The Golden Rules of Drug Use

The Golden Rules of Drug Use

AUTHOR

GRANT TAYLOR KINION

EDITORS

M.L.P. and R.A.K.

PUBLISHER

ROLLED PAPERS PUBLISHING LTD.

The Golden Rules of Drug Use
by Grant Taylor Kinion

First Published Oct. 2025 in Montrose, Colorado, United States of America

The Golden Rules of Drug Use
Published by Rolled Papers Publishing Ltd.
PO Box 3511
Montrose, CO 81402
United States
TheGRODU@gmail.com

eBook ISBN: 979-8-9936713-0-7
Paperback ISBN: 979-8-9936713-1-4
Library of Congress Control Number: 2025923669

DISCLOSURE: The stories in this book are true. As such, the names have been changed to protect the identities of any individual that may have played a part in these stories except for mine. I felt what I have to say is too important to hide behind a pseudonym. Any reader should know and understand that I am not a medical provider. As such my book is not to be taken as medical advice. These are my opinions that have formed as a direct result from my experiences while being a medical patient. Everything in my book is only meant to point out some existing problems, help create new discussions, and present better solutions.

Dedications

-First and foremost, dedicated to my mother. Who never let me go through anything with my eyes shut. Thank you for teaching me perspective.

-Dedicated to Mrs. McD, who on day one of 6th Grade English made the entire class promise that if any of us were ever published we would dedicate our first book to her, no matter what the literary subject was. If she hadn't been such an exceptional teacher, none of us would have.

-Also dedicated to one of my closest friends, R.A.K. who was the sole motivating force behind me starting and finishing this book when he said, "...you seem like a guy who can get things done to me." And we weren't even talking about writing a book. Thank you for lighting a fire under my ass with honest-to-God good old-fashioned encouragement.

-Last, but not least, dedicated to my oldest childhood friend who went through so many of these adventures with me and more. You kept me grounded for a great many years. Thank you for helping me learn modesty and humility.

Introduction

Why write a book? Or rather why even try? I'm undereducated, underworked, underpaid, underappreciated, undermined, and misunderstood. I've never been someone who was well spoken in the moment. You know, the moment when you need or even just want to sound like you've got it together? Or simply show that you are in fact intelligent? In those moments my brain sends my thoughts to the back of my throat, where they trip over my tongue and slam into the back of my teeth before stumbling out of my mouth, incomplete, jumbled, and usually partial. The more I talk the worse it gets. And that is usually the best-case scenario for me. Like an automobile pile-up, only it was my words crashing into the back of my teeth. Like a contortionist acrobat's first day at circus school. On paper it is a bit easier for me to communicate clearly. With a basic understanding of one's native language, I believe most can be clear and concise, or at least more so in writing or print than verbally. As long as it is legible, how can you not be? When you can write it down, review it, edit it, rewrite it again, and repeat until it says exactly what you meant to convey and how you meant to convey it. When I'm engrossed in a conversation with a friend or especially a newer acquaintance, I rarely get my opinions and thoughts out correctly. When I do, as I said, it's usually incorrect or incomplete at best. I imagine it is the same for the other party involved in a conversation. Things, especially life, moves too fast these days. So, this book or books, however many I end up writing, are an unheard side of the story. Unconsidered and unconventional solutions from a perspective that hasn't been considered, even if it should have been from the very start. It is for that reason it is important to keep an open mind and read the entire book with open eyes, and a clear mind.

I'm writing this book first, and in particular because we've all heard from the medical professionals, current, retired, and "experts" in their fields. We've all heard from various politicians and their unrealistic plans for combating drugs and illegal drug use. We've heard from current and former law enforcement about how to solve the fentanyl crisis and win the war on drugs. And we've even heard from current and former addicts as well, even loved ones who have lost a relative to an addiction or overdose about how to avoid and prevent travesties like these accidental deaths. But we have never heard from a current medical patient who has achieved quality of life through proper utilization of not only medical marijuana, but of potentially harmful and supposedly highly addictive medication as well. Personally, I have to ask, "if I can do it the right way and not have a problem, is there really a reason why others can't?"

So that's where I decided to start…Somewhere familiar, somewhere there's a sore spot that is constantly being thrown in our faces. Somewhere there is great misunderstanding especially by those who try to politicize them and those who profit from them...Drugs.

Almost everyone who doesn't do, or never has done drugs, misunderstands them. Almost everyone that does drugs also misunderstands them. Most medical providers who prescribe drugs only understand them from a thirdhand education about the chemical's standpoint, rarely a firsthand accounting of what these sensations, side effects, or the actual intoxication of the drugs themselves, feels like. Let alone what being addicted is. But I do.

TABLE OF CONTENTS:

An Unconventional Origin Story

I was born into a financially stable family. Far from rich, not poor either, simply a comfortable middle-class family (when there still was a strong middle class) from a rural farming community, in a still small hidden pocket of the U.S.A. My family structure eventually turned into a low income, single parent family shortly after my mother divorced my abusive alcoholic father during my early childhood. One event out of many that led to that, an overnight standoff with the cops after a wild night at our local Alcoholics United Club. Doesn't really matter which one, they're all the same, pseudo-elitist members only bars, that hide behind the veil of philanthropy. Loosely represented by some noble member of the animal kingdom or another, but in reality they are just a modern-day Speakeasy. It was June 2nd, 1988, and I was eight years old.

The story landed on the front page of our small town's local newspaper the next morning, but not the headline. It was just to the right of the headline, it was the second article after the main story, and it detailed how My father barricaded himself inside my childhood home for 14 hours before eventually surrendering to his attorney. It talked about how the incident began with two shots fired into the air. The truth is that the two shots in the air were in the middle of a domestic disturbance which was the actual big bang to that nightmare. Going out and drinking too much in the first place was just my father's way of lighting the fuse. It explained how my few country neighbors were evacuated, including my childhood best friend who happened to also be my closest next-door neighbor at the time. And how the sheriff and deputies at the time spent the evening trying to talk him out. At one point dear old dad even turned his phone off and over to his business' answering service. I would've loved to be a fly on the wall when the sheriff tried to call him back and instead got some poor unsuspecting schmuck who had no idea what was going on and wasn't even there.

I also would've loved to include the actual article in my book, verbatim, but I was afraid it would violate copyright infringement and further delay my book, so I made an executive decision to prioritize getting my message out there. Perhaps it'll leave something special for a possible future hardback edition. In any case, that was essentially what the article said in our local paper, the morning after my father decided to be a Redneck Rambo and have a standoff with the cops. There was one sentence that more or less stated that after the standoff began my father barricaded himself inside the house after his wife and son got out safely. And it could not have been more understated or downplayed. There was a whole other story that led to that incident, but I suppose there always is. At least two other articles followed in future weeks of printings of our local small-town newspaper. In short, he managed to get his charges reduced to 18-9-119 (4) Failure or refusal to leave premises or property upon request of a peace officer (H-1) as filed on June 6th, 1988. It resulted in a fine, time served, alcohol classes, and therapy. A lot of good that light handed slap on the wrist did.

That was one, out of many events that led my mother to eventually divorce my father about three years later, and who can blame her? That standoff, and all the other moments of depravity that add up and lead to something like a standoff, from someone with an alcohol problem on that level, for fifteen years. Not to mention all the hell he put me, his own son, through with plenty of trauma and abuse. All roads led her to divorce him and also caused him to lose his family more than once. After that, it was only my mother and I most of the time. Aside from my occasional visits, weekend stayovers, and further abusive moments with and from "him." Back then I honestly believed that alcohol, any amount, even the smallest drop, would turn me into a monster, as it did him. As if it were some magical instant asshole potion. And for honesty's sake, for some people, it is. But for most of us, you don't have to let it be something bad. One of my favorite Benjamin Franklin quotes is, "Beer is proof that God loves us and wants us to be happy." I even had a tee shirt that featured that exact quote. But why does it end so badly for so many? That's another reason why I'm writing this book. It simply doesn't have to be that way.

High school psychology 101 and health classes from the sixth grade to the twelfth, along with the DARE program, all said if someone, like me, grows up in a house with an addict, the likelihood of that person also becoming an addict is exponentially higher. If there are more than one individual in that household or even in the immediate or extended family that overindulges in recreational substances, the potential to develop an addiction or substance abuse increases. Add some serious trauma to that and it's like adding a multiplier to the percentage possibility of that person becoming an addict. I will tell you that if that were one hundred percent true, I wouldn't have been able to write all this after I discovered it, let alone been able to discover it. The reality is becoming and staying an addict is far more of a choice than a lot of people are willing to admit. You simply don't let something like being told it is inevitable that you will be an addict, turn you into one.

When I started working, I started working for free. That's the real ground floor. Helping my best friend's family at eight-years-old and on. I was taught that the only payment I should expect from them is gratitude and be thrilled if it came with a hot meal. His family was in a bad way, and more than financially, so after my parents explained that I was more than happy to help them every chance that I could. When I began working for pay, as a tax paying American at the age of thirteen, I already had a strong work ethic. So, holding down two jobs in the summer, one of which I carried through the school season for years, was no big deal. My year-round job was at a local equipment rental yard. As well as annually returning to my second job, teaching swimming lessons which was, of course, seasonal. I still managed to attend and graduate junior high and high school. In no small part thanks to a promise I made to an ex-girlfriend, to get my high school diploma.

Following high school, I shared a two-bedroom apartment with one of my oldest friends. A short eight months after finding personal freedom as a young adult, I was evicted from my first apartment for smoking marijuana, as was my roommate and close friend. I ended up homeless for a little over a year. He found residency a lot sooner than I did. Weed was still all-the-way-illegal and illegal in all fifty states as marijuana prohibitionists were still controlling the narrative with a nearly one-hundred-year iron grip on marijuana rhetoric. "Marijuana is a gateway drug." As time went on, they would eventually and simultaneously try to convince everyone that there is no difference between weed, cocaine, heroin, meth, or any other street drugs. I always pictured rhetoric like that, being cooked up by fat rich people with too much money and power sitting around a long imposing square wooden table, each with an alcoholic beverage in one hand and a tobacco pipe, cigarette, or cigar in the other, and liquor driven felonies like one or two DUIs under their belts, sometimes even accompanied by domestic violence where alcohol "may" have been a factor.

Anyway, after spending a little over a year being homeless, I finally got hungry enough and fed up enough that I quit smoking pot, cleaned my system out in two weeks so I could pass a UA, which I did, to get a job climbing communication towers for the next three years. After a few more accidents, and in an even more dangerous industry than my previous run of the mill construction jobs, I realized that particularly dangerous employment meant certain disability, death, and/or dismemberment. So, I sought a different type of employment. I ended up going from being an extreme construction worker four-hundred feet in the air, to a desk jockey as a front desk receptionist at a medical clinic. I traded my tool belt and safety harness for a keyboard, a desk phone, and purple scrubs (their company uniform color). My skinny ass looked like an anorexic Barney impersonator in my royal purple Dickies brand scrubs, and we all hate Barney. (It was that damn song!) But at least I had dodged a bullet and avoided becoming disabled and an early death, or so I thought.

At that point in my life, I had already been in more car accidents and had more work injuries than most people do in their entire lives. Few were severe, all were accumulative. The doctor I worked in purple scrubs for was in chronic pain himself and very quickly recognized that I too was suffering with a lot of pain. It takes one to know one. I can say it was a distinct advantage for him to be able to help me. That mutual understanding by a shared experience. That has become more, and more of an apparent disadvantage, the more I see medical providers who not only lack that perspective from personal experience but are nearly completely healthy. This was also around the time I started having these weird neurological events and severe migraines. If you have never had a severe migraine, and in case you have an incorrect impression about what a severe migraine is, like I did, and so you don't have to find out the hard way, like I did, migraines are one of the worst things a human being can experience and endure. Being a decent man and a dedicated medical professional, the doctor I worked for tried to help me. For the most part, he did. Then I was hit two more times with two more car accidents that made all of my symptoms and ailments so much worse. It was equal to the small pebbles that start a large rockslide. The Doctor I worked for referred me to his good friend, as well as his personal medical care provider, with the caveat that I would get the grade A level doctor fellowship treatments and prices, which, by the way, is top level care at cost and don't let them bullshit you, of course they scratch each other's backs.

That was when I went from sober and hurt, to feeling way more pain and being so over medicated that sobriety was a delusion. At twenty-six years old, I was on thirteen different prescription medications, plus the over-the-counter medications I was already taking to survive the injuries I had accumulated from the age of seventeen to twenty-six. Even though I still wasn't taking any recreational drugs anymore, including alcohol and tobacco, I was also the furthest from sober that I have ever been. All by following my doctor's orders and telling him everything, a full disclosure scenario. During my rearing years, I was taught that you needed to be honest with your family physician no matter what. That they have your best interest in mind. But what happens when your medical providers are not only getting your medication from corporate pharmaceutical manufactures but their education as well? That's right, I asked what happens when the drug manufacturers also educate our medical professionals? Trick question, nothing happens, well nothing good anyway.

You get overly doped up and it may have already happened. And then you lose all viable herbal and homeopathic cures and treatments as they weren't all snake oil, but they're now seen only as snake oil. Profit draining snake oil.

But what about our European brethren? Rumor has it that European doctors not only have the education to prescribe prescription medications but the education to prescribe herbal treatments, along with the interactions herbal and natural remedies have with prescriptions medications. It seems to be more advantageous to utilize both worlds instead of simply relying on chemically compounded medications.

So what qualifies me to give this advice? I survived. Just kidding, but only sort of kidding. Perspective from experience is step number one for giving any advice. That is only one part of the reason, but an obviously crucial part of it. After all, will you take advice from someone with no experience, or the guy with so much experience he's not only seen and been on both sides, but it could be argued he's a convert of sorts. Someone who is made to be a believer, so to speak, by personal experiences.

I was a part of year one of First Lady Nancy Reagan's D.A.R.E. program in the fifth grade. The guinea pig class. Our own smalltown sheriff taught our D.A.R.E. class along with the other fifth grade classes for the other four small local elementary schools in Montrose County. As it was for the rest of the country as well. Before he said a word, he drew a horizontal line all the way across the blackboard, approximately in the middle, dividing it into a top and bottom half. "Good morning. For those of you who don't know me, I'm your local Sheriff, Dean Bill. I'm here to speak to you about the D.A.R.E program. You and all the other fifth grade classes across the nation are the first to do this program, and I'll be teaching it to all five elementary schools in our county." He went to a different elementary school each day of the week. Ours was on Fridays. "The first time you get high will be the most wonderful thing you will ever experience, after that you're hooked." He said, as he drew a large fast arc that started on the far left side of the line he drew halfway up the chalkboard (the normal starting point). He drew it slightly diagonally but mostly angled upwards and a little to the right all the way to the top of the blackboard where it apexed in an arch and then went sharply downward with a slight diagonal direction a little further still to the right, ending slightly lower than the line that traversed the middle of the board. As he drew this first arch, he explained, "After you've gotten high and stayed high for a few hours (the apex of the arch) then you come down (the sharp downward slant). But you come down so hard that you end up feeling worse than you did before you got high." The horizontal line, representing a normal/healthy state of mind and body and the sheriff coming to a dramatic brief pause, when he continued. "You then spend the rest of your life trying to reach that ultimate unobtainable high again. Each time you take a drug, any drug, you won't get as high as you did the first time. Every time you get high, your high will be a lower high than the time before. And each time when you come down off any drug, you will feel sicker, and sicker, and sicker." As he dramatically drew another sharp arch, after sharp arch, after sharp arch. Each one reaches a slightly lower elevated apex of height on the board, than the previous arch. The subsequent arches ended by dipping lower, and lower below the normal line and ending lower, and lower than the previous arch on the bottom of the board until the entirety of the arches, even the high parts, were further, and further under the normal line. "Until you end up trying to get high, just to feel a little less sick." The beginning of the DARE program, the first of many generalizations, lies, exaggerations, and miseducations.

Look, we know that is what it is like on heroin, sort of, you still get high, just sicker, and sicker after each time that you do, and the high is supposedly less, and less, but would anyone continue to do something that only made them feel worse? No, that's why things like heroin and fentanyl actually do continue to get you high, but they simultaneously ruin your physical and mental health, and faster than most other recreational substances, making you simultaneously sicker, and sicker without it. This was a generalization across the board about all recreational drugs, including marijuana, and a huge misconception.

Less than half a decade later, during what was a brand-new rave scene, the rhetoric was "If you do ecstasy, you will deplete your serotonin supply, and you will never be happy again." Now they are using MDMA, aka Ecstasy, for rather successful therapy with sexual assault victims and PTSD patients among others. And in case you didn't know, you cannot deplete your supply of serotonin. It is something your body normally makes on a regular basis, as long as everything is copacetic. I'm not saying ecstasy is safe. I'm saying it may not be the demon it was made out to be either.

After witnessing what alcohol did to my father, completing D.A.R.E. (and graduating from the program with honors), and still being a young ignorant child, I made a lot of jokes about people being doped up, when someone would do something stupid, made a mistake, or I was trying to jostle someone a bit. Over the years I've surmised that it's probably why my seventh-grade health teacher, when assigning report subjects, assigned me medical marijuana, as a school report. At first, I was appalled. I didn't want to do a report on "the devil's grass" as I was sure that marijuana, or any drug, had no real value, let alone medicinal value or use. And at around thirteen-years-old, fresh out of "DO NOT DO DRUGS FOR ANY REASON," school, along with four years before that, was Bruce's flip out. I simply couldn't imagine that anything would change my mind about dope or alcohol.

I took the report I was assigned, as I felt like I had no choice. Begrudgingly, I began the legwork of researching my report subject. I was almost immediately beyond shocked, to discover the various medical uses of something I was taught was so horrible, by someone I was always taught and told could be trusted, an officer of the law. Not only an officer of the law, but the sheriff of our small town. It may as well have been Andy Griffith himself who taught the D.A.R.E. program. To top that off, promoted by the First Lady herself! Who as a little kid wouldn't trust the information in a program like that? Not to mention that not too long before this, I watched my grandfather die a horrible death from bladder cancer because of tobacco use. You can imagine my initial feeling of possible betrayal when I find out, at least marijuana, is not the demon it was made out to be, but it even could have at least eased his suffering. And I learned it from three different books in that little middle school library. My simple middle school research, in our simple country school library, showed me there were options. Not only where the medical field and government claim nothing but hopeless and dire situations from drug use, especially at the time, but options where I was taught there was nothing but fleeting bliss, followed only by ever increasing and horrible travesties. How could this be?

Soon after that, I learned an even different perspective by reading about the hippies. Make love not war, feel good, protesting social injustice, 1960's hippies. The Chicago Seven's Jerry Rubin's Just Do It and Abbie Hoffman's Woodstock Nation. Two books that piqued my curiosity from two characters that shall we say, at the least, had a checkered and colorful past, depending on your perspective. In their books they described smoking marijuana and how enlightening it was, and how hard it was to procure, and how "The Man" was really lying about it and other things. And they wrote about tripping acid, and eating hallucinogenic mushrooms, and protesting for a cause, among other things. They preached that the mere act of doing drugs was the kind of protest and defiance necessary to progress mankind and open everyone's mind. I admit, I was curious even if I've never been quite so antiestablishment as they were. And it turns out they were mostly correct. About the drugs, not about burning a city down. And they would've been even more correct if not for the scourge that hardcore street drugs would cause. Make no mistake, the 1960s wasn't only about the wonders and curiosity of, "what does that drug feel like?" It was the idea that war, hate, and violence weren't a necessary thing anymore. And moving past those barriers was and is the next necessary step to true equality. That you could open your mind and expand your perception with the assistance of drugs (F.Y.I. also possible without drugs and more so in many ways), opening yourself up to the different realms of possibilities. It was the notion of freedom of expression and what freedom actually is and how freedom isn't free at all. And it's not like in ancient times or at least shouldn't be like Genghis Khan times for example. When violence was life and power, until recent history, century wise.

Now, I have always had a wonderful imagination. One that was so grand, it often got me in trouble while I was daydreaming in class as a child instead of paying attention. And at the same time, it often got me out of trouble with an inventive coyness that few would catch, even today. So, the idea that you could see something that wasn't there, even more so, being able to invoke a controlled hallucination, like plucking characters and even inventions straight from my mind, making them tangible, was an intriguing idea to me.

Fast forward a bit more. To when I tried drugs. Martin Luther King Jr. Day, 1996. I was fifteen and marijuana was my first experience with any recreational drug, alcohol and tobacco included. It is different from person to person, which drug someone tries first, if they try drugs, as well as their experience with that drug. I was hesitant, yet so curious, looking back it seemed inevitable. And it turns out, one of the few true things from D.A.R.E., the first time really was amazing! But that was where most of the similarities ended in that aspect. I felt wonderful, better than I ever had before. My apprehensions, hesitations, and anxieties that all young people feel as they are unsure of themselves were gone, virtually nonexistent. As if I had never experienced the uneasiness of life or the core rattling sensations of personal trauma. My best friend and I smoked what was referred to as Mexican Brick Weed in the small patch of forest behind his property out of a makeshift pipe, improvised from a mechanical brass fitting. After getting high for my first time, his 3rd or 4th, we walked around our own private slice of Lost Boy's paradise. "Second star to the right," Lost Boys. Not the "don't invite them in," Lost Boys.

Some country boys have a favorite fishing hole, some have a favorite hang out at a friend's house, we had our little hundred-acre woods. I'm sure it was smaller than one hundred acres. But I couldn't help put the play-on-words as homage to one of my favorite childhood books and characters. Getting high for the first time didn't seem like a storybook, but it did seem like I was in a movie. Like literally in a movie. Not that creepy feeling you get when you think someone might be watching your every move. More where someone slowed down the frames per-second rate on a movie I was watching. Barely slow enough that I could see it in my vision. The outline black borders of the individual frames, passing vertically upwards, slicing through each frame of my vision. In the series of many individually framed pictures that make pictures into movies, as we walked through the various paths deer, racoons, and who knows what else wandered along before we even existed. It has never been an experience like that again. I don't think I would've wanted it to be, and it wasn't as I was told, that I would want to "chase the dragon," but with weed it would probably be more like "catching a bunny" if it even had that aspect to it. I also never spent any time doing drugs to feel normal again, medical uses aside but reality is even those should probably not be taken with the intent of feeling normal, but better, ironically. If you add a chemical, recreational or prescription, it will always be different. But every time I used drugs recreationally, I have gotten high, every time. Never once did I take them to "get normal." And I never necessarily sought that same high either, again like I was told I would. Sometimes I simply sought the next one. Not necessarily the next drug either, but rather the next experience, the next sensation, for not all sensations can or should be achieved through drugs. There is a line there, and it is one of the lines that gets people going down a bad rabbit hole. For example, do you know eating hot peppers can induce an adrenaline rush? They can also severely damage your taste buds, esophagus, and stomach. So much so that they can put you in the hospital and in some cases even kill you. So, I wouldn't recommend it. But sounds familiar, yes? Similarly, someone can take too much heroin, or speed, or fentanyl, and end up in a worse situation, even if they don't die. Ask those competitive eaters, especially the ones who specialize in hot food contests, when they're old, and have an ulcer in their stomach that's twice the size of their stomach, how that worked out for them in the long run and if they can manage to answer you back, between the handfuls of antacids, generic versions of Prilosec, and Bean-O, I bet they'd say, "it wasn't worth the ten dollar trophy from the trophy store, but at least it's engraved, like my gut." And similar to using hardcore drugs, competitive eating comes with a danger that few of us ever think about. The sensation of never being full, always feeling hungry. Similarly, someone can overdo it with Tylenol, Ibuprofen, working too much, or mixing the wrong cleaning products together. Even though I hadn't fully realized it at the time, lots of things can hurt you when misused, not just the obvious ones like dope, sharp objects, and bullets. And yet in my personal journeys and experiences, would I end up addicted? Dead? Incarcerated? At that point who really knew. Realistically, it was all on the table of possibilities, the good as much as the bad. I must admit, as far as doing drugs and breaking the law goes, I got lucky. More than a few times, and in more than a few ways. One could even argue that I was being bad the right way, by not taking it all the way. Even though I had many friends who would end up being not so fortunate, walking such a dangerous line. But what an adventure of unique learning and alternative perspective that it all ended up being. Even the really bad stuff. Because even you will fuck up, in life, and in general. The trick is learning from it.

After trying and liking marijuana, I spent the next five years, my early adulthood, living life like an off-the-clock rockstar, but behind closed doors, and as quietly as possible. But did I ever live! Morrison, Joplin, Hendrix, Garcia, they all would have all been proud and I still managed to hold down a job, at times two or more. No, I'm not referring to any kind of illegal hustle either, but legit, tax paying work, and I still managed to graduate high school, again, thanks to a certain promise I made to a certain person. Keep in mind drugs were still all illegal then. No safe enlightened states for marijuana, no research into the potential mental health benefits of hallucinogens (even though those of us who were smoking pot, and on occasion tripping hallucinogens, were happier than everybody else, wonder why?). Nope, all of it was illegal, in all fifty states in America, unless you wanted to be a worthless drunk. Which they still lock you up for in certain situations. So, being drunk is legal, yes, but kosher? Seems far from it. Because even an intoxicant that is legal has limits, a line that you don't cross. Most things do. In the past very few ever sought to ask the question, or even considered, could hallucinogens and other street drugs have a medicinal purpose? Like I said, except for those who used them.

One day some friends and I were smoking a little pot, and conversating in my apartment while we got down, playing some video games. When one of our friends that we called "Cowboy" volunteered to buy some beer. So, he and my oldest friend Sonny headed out to the liquor store, while I stayed behind to man the fort. About the time they should've been back from beer retrieval, I heard some conversing in the breezeway between the apartments, which was unusual, so I went to the peephole in the front door to take a look.

All I could see was a crescent shaped slivered edge of a magnified thumb print on the border of the peephole glass. The bulk of the print was mostly shaded from being pressed against the glass on the peephole, but one side of the thumb was partially raised, failing to completely cover the glass on the peephole from the outside of the door, which barely let enough light onto the edge of his thumb to see the ridges and valleys that make every finger and thumb print unique. It must have been the same perspective small bugs and insects have of a human thumb right before meeting an untimely demise as they get smashed, which was ironic because as soon as I realized it was a thumb covering up the peephole, I also realized it was the thumb of the law, or rather of a law enforcement officer. Which made me feel very small, like a bug about to be squashed, hence the ironic part.

Knowing it was the police and knowing a little of my own state's law, that without a warrant or good probable cause to look "further," it is little more than clear and present sight only, and if they didn't find anything in the apartment, they couldn't search me. Very quietly and quickly, I gathered everything I had that was illicit or could warrant (yes, pun intended) a deeper search, and either put it in my pockets or hid it so well that it was far beyond out in the open so as to avoid clear and present sight, thus nothing could give any probable cause. I waited, directly on the other side of my apartment's front door, for that inevitable heavy-handed knock that makes lawbreakers', drug users', and even law-abiding citizens' hearts alike, skip a beat. And sure enough, shortly after that…

A "BAM, BAM, BAM," came rapping at my front door! (A little shout out to one of my favorite poets) "Police depa…"

I didn't give him a chance to finish as I popped the door open. "Hello officers." I said to the three of them all standing proud in the apartment breezeway, clad in the dark blue garments and metallic equipment that makes a Montrose City Police Officer's uniform.

"We received a call complaining about the smell of marijuana. May I please have your name?" Asked Officer Amada, not the first time I had dealt with him. I gave Officer Amada my name and one of his cohorts repeated my last name with a queried tone, "Kinion?" He followed by, "Are you Bruce's son?"

Hanging my head a little bit, "Yeah, but don't worry, I hate him too." Something I would usually say out of default to anyone in my small hometown who would disapprovingly ask if I was Bruce's unholy offspring. It was simply a defensive way to protect myself, by hopefully putting a little distance between him and I, and also a way of indicating that whatever he did to them, I received worse.

"I didn't say that." The same officer abruptly replied.

"You didn't have to. I know what he did." I responded with resolve.

"Regardless, we know it's you who is smoking marijuana, and we know because you tried to cover it up with Lysol, the whole common stairwell reeks of it, we can smell it."

Having recently lost my job to an employer who cared less about life and more about his cocaine when he was let off from being on probation (something he didn't disclose to me anytime during my employment or interview for the job.) He continued to make money solely to do more blow and it eventually caught up to him and became a worse situation. But it still left me laid off and with my roommate who was between construction contracts himself. We didn't even have the money for dish detergent, let alone brand name air freshener or sanitizer like Lysol, and it showed. "Officers, I can't even afford cleaning supplies, let alone Lysol." As I opened my door further, with the same arm gesture Vana White uses to reveal a vowel. Emphasizing the mountain of uncleaned dishes in the kitchen burying the sink under a heaping pile of porcelain, plastic dishes, and cups alike, each cultivating its own unique brand of filth, disgust, and even a variety of mold.

"Good point." Said Officer Amada. "We still know it was you that has been smoking pot."

"Well, somebody doesn't like the smell of it!" Exclaimed one of the other officers, interjecting his two cents.

"I just finished the remainder of a roach. It was all I had." I said with a bold poker face. Lying my ass off with a quarter ounce or so of some 90s dank laying in the bottom of my pocket, cuddling my handblown glass pipe. And I know what you're thinking, how does someone recently unemployed afford weed? The answer, I had already bought it before I was laid off and street drugs in general typically have an "all sales are final," and "no returns, no refunds," business policies.

"Where's the rest of the roach then?"

"I ate it." I promptly responded, quickly firing back with the same bold look on my poker face, expressing that was the obvious course of action. At one time, it was an old school hippie tradition. "It's what you do with a roach," I stated. But seriously people, that's too far. Don't eat your roaches, that's gross. And a tradition that should've been dead and gone a long time ago.

Officer Amada sighs, "will you give us permission to look around."

"Do I have a choice?" I asked as I shrugged my shoulders, already knowing full well that I did not.

"Yeah, you can absolutely say no." Amada pauses for a brief second, "but then we'll just go get a warrant and search your apartment anyway."

What choice did I have? I opened the door, gestured welcome in, and gave them the go ahead, as I said, already knowing their search would be fairly limited to clear and present sight only which, once again, limited their ability to gaze deeper. That is as long as they didn't see anything that would give probable cause. (Learn your laws. If not for this reason, so that you at least know exactly what line(s) you are crossing.)

The three of them began looking around and after a while of not finding anything, one leaned over to another and whispered in a volume barely under a normal conversation, but loud enough that I heard him, "He's got it on him." I couldn't help it, I cracked a shit eating grin, because he was right. I knew it and they knew it. We all knew it, and there was nothing any of them could do about it. After searching for about 30 minutes and realizing they couldn't search further without violating my rights, they left without being able to even write a citation for misdemeanor possession, let alone finding probable cause to search further.

A few minutes after that, my cowardly prick of a landlord shows up and hands me a thirty-day eviction notice. He coldly pounded on the door, I opened it, he handed the eviction notice to me and quickly turned and scurried away, with his hairless shriveled balls between his legs. Not even a single word of human decency or sign of remorse. That's okay, he was a slumlord anyway. When my roommate arrived back at our mutual dwelling, we talked and decided to bail. We moved all our stuff to a relative's storage unit and friends' houses. And threw the rest away that we either couldn't find a home for or wasn't worth keeping. We told ourselves and our friends and families that we decided not to waste money on rent and live in our cars for a while until we could figure something else out so we could save up some money. But that wasn't reality.

Maybe it was out of pride, maybe it was not wanting pity, or not wanting people to know we had failed at being on our own so quickly. It didn't really matter. The reality was, we had no money for first month rent, last month rent, and a damage deposit. Not individually or together. So, we couldn't have rented another place, even if we wanted to. If we had stayed in the apartment for the next thirty days, until the end of our eviction notice we only would've incurred more debt with the utilities, because as I mentioned we were both struggling to find steady, quality employment. Our small, still undiscovered hidden gem of a farm town hadn't become vibrant yet and there was very little work, hence no money. But Montrose would eventually blossom, much to everyone's dismay, who grew up here in the 1980s and early 1990s, but especially mine. It was kind of like watching Mayberry turn into Reno, seemingly overnight, but with zero casinos.

I spent the next year and some change being and experiencing varying degrees of homelessness. Whether it was by choice, out of denial, or maybe it was out of stubbornness for keeping my independence, it didn't really matter how or why at that point. I simply was homeless. I went from sleeping in my vehicle, to sleeping in a broken-down hunting camper, heated by an electric heater on the end of an one-hundred-foot extension cord, to eventually sort of squatting. I say sort of squatting because I had the permission of the current/former owner, the bank simply hadn't finished the foreclosure on it yet and hence hadn't taken possession. So at least I was coming up in some way, shape, or form. Until finally, I was tired and hungry enough to want a better life. So much so that I stopped smoking pot, cleaned my system out in two weeks with detox tea, water, mountain dew, and sweating my ass off in Epsom salt soaks. All so I could take and pass a U.A., and then I could start what I thought would be a decent, quality job that could change my life for the better. It wasn't. But if you want a quality job without a college degree, requirement number one: You must be able to pass an U.A. (Urine Analysis), drug screening. And yeah, I could've cheated it or tried to, but if you do that, then you have to cheat the next one, and the one after that, and then the unexpected surprise random U.A., or the dreaded "when you get injured on the job," U.A. Let's see you use someone else's pee out of a fake bladder with one or both arms in slings or casts. Or while you're on your way to the hospital in the back of an ambulance or taken from you by catheter in the ER while you are unconscious. Good thing you managed to safely keep and store human urine, that doesn't belong to you, in the back of your freezer, next to that frozen pot roast that's in the queue for next Tuesday's family dinner. Ever wonder how your family felt about a stranger's urine being frozen and stored in the deep freezer next to the family food? Did they even know? Ahh, what they don't know can't hurt them or at least if it does, they'll never know why, right?

When you flunk that UA after you were hurt, your medical bills don't get covered because they claim you were high on the job, even if you weren't. And only because it was in your system, they assume that's why your injury happened. It's not fair, but it is the law. Even though it takes days, weeks, and sometimes a month or longer for a lot of substances to leave your system. So much for, innocent until proven guilty. Maybe it should be innocent until you mess up, then we'll assume guilt to keep from doing the right thing, which will save us money at your expense. It's one of those inequities that science will one day fix so they can accurately tell if you were currently under the influence, and not the remaining traces of substances from a fun evening of partying. But until it does, the point is cheating so you can get high is a fleeting victory, sooner or later everyone gets caught. Because sometimes, if you don't have a degree from a college, you have to risk your life to make good money. It was that kind of job that I found. It was unfortunately not those kind of good paying, appreciative employers.

The U.A. I took was for employment with a communication tower company. They'll hire anyone who has the balls to climb a tower for barely over minimum wage and can pee clean at least once. Already accustomed to shit pay, even from my own father, I was just that asshole they were looking to take advantage of. Ironically and in hindsight, that work was just what I needed at twenty years old. Minus the twelve dollars an hour part, for what would soon become listed as one of the most dangerous jobs in the world. That was low pay, for most jobs, but especially for a dangerous one. It probably wasn't recognized as such a dangerous profession at that point due to shady business practices of screwing your employees over so you can keep your insurance rates low. It's just the lives of poor people. Let's get those telecommunication towers and antennas up and running, we have got to advance technology at any expense. Cell phones are important, money and profit, even more so. (Please note my intended sarcasm). And know, this is not conjecture, as they did it to me.

Turns out the part they teach you in school (and in D.A.R.E.) about the developing brain being hindered by taking any mind-altering substance (that includes alcohol) before the age of twenty-eight had some truth to it. Dead sober, and believe it or not, enjoying life and enjoying the experience of being alive and going to work, it seemed like I was more than maturing. I was evolving, I was catching up, and even surpassing my peers, associates, friends, and family. I noticed I could handle stressful events that before I would have handled like a child throwing a temper tantrum. Now I handled them as a reasonable adult should. My patience grew, my ignorance, and arrogance shrank, as I began to become the man I was meant to be. The quote goes, "When I was a child, I played as a child, I thought as a child, I acted as a child. When I became a man, I put away childish things." Where climbing towers was an exciting and adventurous once-in-a-lifetime experience, few people get to do, it was also very dangerous work. And it wasn't long before a series of unfortunate events made me rethink that particular career choice.

I'm no stranger to injuries. As a matter of fact, and by default, I'm a bit of a pro. Sort of a practice makes perfect, scenario. But I never intended to practice anything like that, so we'll simply call them accidents, because that is what they were, unintentional accidents. A shit-ton of unintentional accidents. But my tons of accidents also led to some heavy perspectives. So much "perspective," that before I was climbing towers, I was already taking handfuls of over-the-counter pain medications, just to make it through the workday and to be able to sleep through the night. All so I could manage to go back to work the next day. Tylenol, Ibuprofen, and Excedrin (The working man's Viagra, because it helps us, the blue collared, get it done). And the PM versions of Tylenol and Ibuprofen for sleep most nights.

Then, while climbing communication towers for a living, I took a blow to the head that involved a three-inch wide, fifteen-foot long, galvanized steel pipe that followed my forehead to the ground, from the top of a truck rack. That I tried and obviously failed to load. Seven stitches, three on the bridge of my broken nose, four above the inside thick fluffy part of my right eyebrow, a concussion, and one hell of a headache. And even though that pipe failed to knock me out, that round went to the large zinc coated steel pipe, by points alone. I honestly never saw the hit coming. Like almost everybody that stepped in the ring with Mike Tyson, but again without a knockout. The next day my dickhead employer challenged my manhood, which I now admit, I let my ego feed into. But that also wasn't my first, or last head injury that came with a complimentary side order of concussion.

"Your crew is driving back to Kansas City tomorrow, so I guess we'll see what kind of man you are." His arrogant ass said, tauntingly. I was not only the first one there, onsite, and ready to roll out that next morning, like every morning, I did it with a smile on my face. Unlike every morning before that, I also did it with two black eyes, a broken swollen and sore nose, a concussion, and one hell of a headache that one of the worst that I have ever had at that point. I drove a full-size F-350 with a sixteen-foot fully loaded winch trailer for a little over twelve hours. From Colorado Springs, CO to Lee's Summit, MO, fudging DOT (Department of Transportation) records, at the direction of the higher-ups at the tower company I worked for, to "do whatever you have to, just haul ass back to home base."

An emergency room visit confirmed my concussion the night before. Which ended with the doctor saying, "don't go to sleep for the next twenty-four hours." To experiencing the entirety of the west to east mind-numbing landscape of Kansas, or as I call it, Flatland with cows. And in case you're wondering, it is exactly the same landscape as the north to south tour of Kansas, west to east is just longer. From Colorado to Missouri, behind the wheel of a DOT certified work truck and trailer sporting one of the biggest, straight out of hell headaches I have ever had at that point in my life, and I had that headache since the steel pipe found my head a little less than twenty-four hours earlier.

About eight months after that, I got my right hand caught in between a winch's metal cable and pulley after my crew left me alone at the top of a tower to de-rig a boom arm by myself. Our crew was tasked with mounting three, fifteen-foot-tall omni antennas to the top of a communication tower. On this particular job, that meant first mounting a temporary forty-foot tower (or boom arm) to the top of the tower. When the headache balls, one or both, got caught on a supporting crossbeam on the way back up the middle of the tower,

I quickly slapped the cable to give it a quick shake so that a vibrational wave would surf down the cable and pop it off the supporting beam, or whatever it was caught on. It popped right off alright, but the tension was so much the cable quickly grabbed my hand by snagging the brown fabric of my brown jersey work glove, like industrial strength Velcro, when it jumped a good length of cable through due to the tension release, instantly pulled my fingers on my right hand into the pulley, pinching them between the cable and the pulley in an unforgiving steel grip.

On one end of the metal cable, the same winch I hauled from Colorado to Missouri, only now I'm four-hundred feet up on a tower, looking at my hand going under the cable, pinched between the pulley and the cable. The cable came to a conclusion at the winch, wrapping around a cable drum, four-hundred feet down to the ground on one side of the pulley, and about three-hundred-sixty feet of cable on the other side (give or take) of the pulley that goes down to two eighty pound headache balls and the load, the equipment for derigging, and a fresh radio. My fingers were clasped in a way that would've made M.C Escher and Houdini jealous. Seemingly disappearing, like an illusion or a magic trick, under the cable, looking like they weren't there at all. It appeared as though my fingers never disrupted the contact between the cable and the pulley. As if all my fingers just freakishly reappeared on the other side of the pulley and cable, again, without disrupting the tangible contact of the two metal parts of basic mechanics. Where my four fingers emerged on the other side of the cable, each one going their own way like the little piggies that went to the market, and then they decided they'd all do their respective individual tasks. Only all of my fingers were crying wee, wee, wee, as I was certain that I wasn't going to take any of my fingers home, and I was kissing them goodbye, almost literally. Even though it looked like a magic trick, it felt like the third level of hell. So strange, as it looked as if the pulley and cable shared no space or consideration for my fingers in between them. My fingers magically reappeared, coming out the other side. All four reaching in four different contorted directions. As if my fingers slipped through an interdimensional doorway that somehow allowed my fingers to escape to the other side. And I would've believed that too, had it not been the next level pain that I had been introduced to.

Thoughts about how the OSHA and CommTrain Class (Communication Tower Climbing Safety Class) taught us, this is how you lose your digits, and your friends now call you "Stumpy," for the rest of your life. If not to your face, then at least behind your back. It only takes seven pounds of pressure to sever a finger from your hand. Seven-hundred-sixty feet of winch cable at five pounds per two feet is nineteen-hundred pounds. With two eighty-pound headache balls plus the derigging equipment, about another forty pounds, equals an approximate, yet cool two-thousand-two-hundred pounds give or take, but when you're talking about losing your fingers, or anything else, nobody gives a shit about any give or take, especially physics. One metric ton of weight, being pulled by a ten-thousand pound lifting capacity winch, that was all clasping me in place, with that massive weight sitting on my fingers, while simultaneously trying to yank my fingers, hell, felt like my whole arm, through the tiny hole on the metal pulley, that held and ran a 5/8th of inch steel cable through it, so it could be smoothly be pulled up and down the inside of that four-hundred-foot tall, self-supported, communication tower.

At that time in my life, I considered myself agnostic. I didn't really believe in anything, yet I hadn't drawn a hardline that there was nothing either. In my childhood I was raised, going to church every Sunday. I even graduated from Sunday School, and I have a commemorative bible to prove it. But at that point, in my early twenties, with everything I had already seen and experienced, I did not and could not believe in anything. Nothing but the ugliness of mankind. No merciful God, no salvation. Religion didn't really make sense to me, but neither did "nothing at all," as Atheists preach. Most people hear a story like this, with an intro like that and think, "let me guess, you cried out to God, and he saved your hand, and you've been a believer ever since, right?"

But you'd be dead wrong. I can honestly say that I wasn't calling out to God. Not out loud, or even in my head, to myself. I was waving my free left arm and hand frantically, trying to get someone's attention, four-hundred feet below me, on the ground while balancing on a cross beam, held frozen in that spot by the grasp of unforgiving steel, waiting to be yanked through the pulley like a cartoon character, only coming out as shredded meat on the other side. As I didn't have a working radio, one was coming up with the derigging equipment. One of my coworkers climbed down with the only good one. He was too lazy to climb back up twenty feet to hand it over to me when he realized it. No, it was much easier for him to climb down three-hundred-eighty feet and send it back up with the derigging equipment. As much movement as I was making to try and get someone to see me, it mattered not as the winch operator and my other six coworkers on the ground couldn't see me. When the pulley and cable grabbed my hand, it also pulled me barely inside the tower's outer edge, out of sight, where I couldn't be seen by the winch operator or anyone else on the ground, making any kind of visual arm signal wasted effort. I was screaming at the top of my lungs, but no one could hear me over the diesel engine of the winch or the four-hundred feet of noise dampening empty air between us. In my head I was kissing goodbye, all the dreams I had about being a glassblower or any kind of artist, or any activity that involved having two fully functional hands, including making proper love to a woman. I was thinking how much life is going to suck for someone whose sole wish in life is to be a craftsman and an artist, to only have a total of four fingers and two thumbs.

My fingers, or something, managed to bog down the winch that had me stuck, screaming for help, even though I was helpless. I was screaming to back the winch up or turn it off, when the winch operator did exactly that. He backed the winch cable up, as to him, it seemed stuck. And it was stuck, bogged down, on my four fingers, that, at the most, gave twenty-eight pounds of resistance against a ten-thousand-pound capacity winch. Keep in mind, ten-thousand pounds is what it will lift safely. In reality it will lift quite a bit more.

When the winch wouldn't move and it instead was strained, bogged down by my four little fingers, and the winch operator finally backed it off a foot or two thinking it was caught on a cross beam on the way up, which it initially most likely was before it briefly broke free, sucking my fingers into near oblivion. The winch operator didn't notice the quick succession of the cable stopping, getting snagged on a supporting cross beam, breaking free, only to quickly choke on my fingers. Only that it had stopped and wouldn't move. When he backed the cable off, my fingers and hand were instantly released from the iron grip of unforgiving machinery as if an enormous metal giant with monstrous strength simply and gently let go, albeit let go too late to avoid any damage. My hand now throbbing, I was certain my fingers, if still attached, were attached by little more than flattened flesh and crushed bone, my fingers, laying in the fabric cradles that my work gloves provided. Like four flesh colored Gumbys barely hanging on to my hand. All four inside of their respective finger sleeves of my brown jersey work glove.

Four-hundred feet up, now freed from my metal aerial trap, I carefully shimmied over to the service ladder on one of the inside corners of the tower. I wrap my right arm around the ladder, attach my chest safety lanyard to the safety cable mounted to the middle of the ladder and I slowly start slinking my way down. Gripping the ladder with my uninjured left hand and hugging the back of the ladder, as if I was hugging a long lost relative, with my right arm, with my right-hand throbbing in intense acute pain. All so I could briefly let go of one ladder rung, to grab the next rung with my left hand, one rung at a time. All the way down the four-hundred-foot tower. Slowly, awkwardly, and painfully, managing to adjust my safety lanyard on the safety cable, around its metal support brackets, every ten feet.

When I reached the ground, the winch operator and my former foreman, Timmy, said, "boy, you better have been hit by lightning."

I lightly chuckled, my eyes shrink wrapped in tears, already knowing full well from previous injuries, the physical and financial setbacks that awaited me. And everything was going so well too. "Close, my hand got caught between the pulley and cable. You guys couldn't see me waving my other arm or hear me yelling for help?"

He gave me a look of shocked devastation, as he had the same safety classes I did. "No. We didn't. I can't see you or anyone near that pulley or the interior equipment. Why didn't you radio down? We need to take your glove off."

"We most certainly do not! And Melvin had the radio." I bluntly hollered back in a firm booming tone and volume.

"Yeah, we need to see how bad it is." Timmy calmly explained.

"Fine but a bad idea." I said as I held out my squashed hand volunteering for some more pain, certain that my digits were loose inside my glove. Slowly and carefully, Timmy inched my brown jersey work glove from my hand. It felt like he was peeling the skin from my hand. Despite that, not only were my fingers attached but they barely looked bruised. And no one was more surprised than me.

When they got me to the hospital, I explained what happened to the emergency room doctor. I explained what the CommTrain Tower Climbing Safety Class and OSHA class both said. That, by all laws of physics, my fingers should not be attached to my hand. They gave me a cup to pee in so I could prove sobriety on the job. See, the dreaded "got hurt on the job" drug test. But after what I told them, I would've insisted on a drug test as well. I managed to fill their drug analysis cup with some fancy one-handed cup, penis, pee juggling. After completing my circus task, they doped me up. For those who believe opioids are all bad, massive pain is unbearable and, in some cases, not this one, unsurvivable. Opioid painkillers changed that. They took a battlefield amputation from an almost certain death sentence to survivable because they weren't going into shock on a hardcore level with the pain at least partially blocked and managed. But we'll get more into that later. At that moment I was simply grateful to have some pain relief.

After almost getting my fingers cleaved off from the sheer force of weight by rounded objects made me think, all night. Not only was I risking my life and health to work on the road for a very minimal amount of money, in a job that is very dangerous. But my employer had already threatened to fire me if I got injured on the job one more time. And that was it, so what was I still doing there? I thought about what happened all night in my Kansas City, MO hotel room. I'd usually watch a movie or two after work to unwind, but that evening I didn't even turn the tv on. I was lost in thought, for hours, sitting on the edge of my hotel bed with a throbbing right hand. How do I still have those fingers? By all rights, I shouldn't. It was a typical Occam's Razor situation. Once all other possibilities have been eliminated, whatever is left, no matter how improbable, is your answer. And I knew, at that moment, a higher power had saved my fingers and hand, had shown me mercy, and had given me a second chance, maybe even a wake-up call as well, and I didn't even need to ask.

The next morning, at continental breakfast, Timmy, the winch operator, showed up at my Lee's Summit, MO hotel. Which was weird, because he lived in Lee's Summit. It was where I was stationed for work, and where our tower company's main corporate headquarters was. Typically, I wouldn't see him until we all gathered at our tower company's office and warehouse at 8:00 or earlier in the morning, to start our day.

"Hey Grant, How's your hand?" asked Timmy.

"Okay, I suppose, considering what could, well, what should have happened." I answered.

He nodded his head in agreement and gave me a grin, acknowledging the bullet I dodged the day before. "Hey bro, just a heads-up but we all had an old coworker, he left a year or two before you came here…he died yesterday." Timmy said sullenly and with the heavy hesitation that comes with near unbearable grief.

"Holy shit Timmy, I am so sorry man. My deepest condolences."

"Thank you for that. He got his climbing harness caught in the cathead." A cathead is a winch designed for rope, and in this case, it was attached to a trailer hitch by welds and mounted in place to the trailer hitch on the back of a work truck. "It pulled him down onto the cathead and foot pedal so he couldn't let off it and he unintentionally asphyxiated himself to death." I gasped at the horror of it all. Dying of asphyxiation is no picnic. But to die of it because you pressed the go pedal, getting your harness stuck in the winch, and thus it pulled you down against the winch and the go pedal as well, making it impossible to release your foot, unable to get off it so it would stop. He must've known that he was helpless and about to die, and there was nothing he or anyone could do. Timmy added, "He only had one coworker with him, and he was one-hundred feet up on a guide tower. By the time he got down to him, it was too late, he was dead. His eyeballs literally hanging out of his head, dead." Not an uncommon occurrence of asphyxiation. "That's why we typically work in four-man crews. Two on the tower, two on the ground. In case anything like that happens." He said, most likely as part of his grieving process, to justify his friend's demise.

I gave Timmy the kind of hug that is only for condolences among men. Hearty, firm, and says, "I'm sorry, keep your chin up, and I'm there for you, brother," all in a tight squeeze with fist clenched, followed by a hearty pat on the back or two. When the brief, but firm, hug came to an end I told him, "Anything I can do for you, you have but to ask, my friend."

"Appreciate that, thank you." He said with gratitude in his voice.

"Unfortunately, that cinches it for me." He looked at me confused, his head partially cocked sideways, as I continued. "After almost losing my digits yesterday, and I should have," He nodded agreeingly as I continued, "I'm done. I need to be. If I keep working at this job, I'm going to end up crippled or worse, dead. In which case, my dreams really are over." Turns out there have been times since when I was almost positive that I had that backwards. Sometimes death seems like a better idea than suffering, especially seemingly endlessly. And if you are suffering yourself, unfortunately you probably know what I mean, and if you're not, you assuredly don't want that firsthand perspective.

"You gotta do what you gotta do. I don't blame you, and I ain't mad 'atcha." Said Timmy.

"Thanks for understanding." I replied.

"And thanks for helping me make up my mind," I thought to myself, not wanting to offend the memory of his recently deceased friend and coworker.

Within the next few days, I was on a plane back home. Having avoided becoming disabled or even dying, simply by changing careers. Turns out, I only thought I was avoiding further physical pain and suffering, as a certain amount of unamicable and unmitigable damage had already been done. At that job, during my variety of previous employment, and previous car accidents. And a minor amount of further damage would eventually put me in an even worse situation, no matter how hard I tried to avoid it.

I moved back to my home state of Colorado, but not my small farm town of Montrose. I temporarily moved in with my mother and grandmother, who themselves, combined households and moved across the state to one of Colorado's big cities, Colorado Springs. At twenty-three years old, having been an employed tax paying American for the last decade, I took a short sabbatical from any kind of work for a few months, then I started looking for a job outside of construction. I ended up finding a small doctor's office that was willing to give my washed-up construction worker ass a chance. I was a part-time front desk receptionist. I ended up being good at it, liking it, and it ended up being perfect for me at the time.

It was perfect because this is when my body began falling apart, seemingly of its own accord, but realistically it was from the accumulation of past injuries and accidents. Sooner or later, your past mistakes catch up with you, injuries especially. Mine sure caught up with me. The doctor I worked for was in chronic pain himself. As such he was able to recognize my agony and tried to help me. Even though I had managed to dramatically change how I made a living with a shift from work that was brutal on the human body, to office work that was more of a brain and social engagement workout than pure physical exertion. Tiring in itself, but an entirely different kind of hard work and exhaustion. This is where I quickly went from being sober and enjoying life on life's terms, despite a vast amount of pain, to scrambling to keep as much quality of life as possible, sobriety be damned. While more, and more, my quality of life started slipping away as my body, my health began a rapid decline. As though I was trying to cradle gallons of water in a desperate embrace without a container, my health slipped away, right through the cracks and crevices of my arms, hands, and fingers, as water would.

I didn't drink alcohol, I didn't smoke pot at that time, and I hadn't even restarted smoking cigarettes again. I was getting through the aches and pains of my days and nights with handfuls of Over-The-Counter pain medications and eventually adding a low-grade muscle relaxer. And then it happened. I was hit two more times, two more car accidents, within two months of each other. Both were the result of someone else being careless and stopping their vehicles by running into mine. While I was courteous enough to stop at two different traffic lights without the assistance of my fellow motorists. Again, I'm kidding. I recognize that shi…accidents happen. Even though both wrecks were on the low end of moderate, a little whiplash, a little concussion, it was all that was needed to take my already spiraling out of control ailments turbo.

I started seeing my boss' good friend, and his personal medical provider, Dr. Horedoor, with my employer's personal referral to handle the car accident stuff. Thinking I had the inside track, and still completely trusting and complacent with doctors, I reported how I felt and the many multiplying symptoms to my medical provider every appointment. And he kept writing me medications. During the ages of twenty-five to twenty-six, I went from three over-the-counter medications and one muscle relaxer to thirteen prescription medications, on top of my three over-the-counter ones. I was higher than most hardcore street addicts get, and on a daily basis, while my doctors are looking at me befuddled and sideways when I would tell them, "I miss being sober."

They'd reply with things like, "why don't you think you're sober?" and "You are sober, as long as you're only taking medications." I can tell you from firsthand experience that is a distinction without any actual difference. Doped up is doped up.

At least a third of the medications he prescribed came with similar caveats. "This medication is typically written for something else entirely, but it has an off-label use as a mood enhancer, pain blocker," or some other supposed surprise benefit. Basically, "off-label use" means that some patients reported improvement where improvement was not expected. Know that drug was never tested for anything other than the intended use. It's kind of like doing cocaine to get through the common cold. It'll probably be the best cold you've ever had without actually taking cold medicine, but the unknown and known risks far outweigh any actual benefit.

When I was over medicated, I described my state of mind at that time, and still do, as "on autopilot." That's downplaying it more than a bit. Basically, that's so fucking high, it's a miracle I was even able wipe my own ass, let alone get everything done that a normal human being can, and should accomplish every day. But somehow, I managed to barely skate by, and with little clear recollection of a fair amount of it. That's so high a homeless street junkie would've been jealous. Ironically, someone can insult me and look down on me, for my prior recreational drug history all they want. I never let it get out of control, and it is the sole reason I was not only able to survive those first eight years of being a ward of the medical community, but I was able to thrive more than most can in a near hopeless situation that the medical field had thrown me into with countless others. And my history is also why I happened to eventually come out on top. Despite some initial losses and setbacks, I was better off for it. Most people without my, or similar, experiences would've wound up addicted, homeless, incarcerated, dead, or any combination thereof.

A year and a half after the last two car crashes, I was more miserable, while being more medicated than most people over the age of fifty, and still in more discomfort than I ever had before, and all by my mid-twenties. I lost my receptionist job of over three years, and hence my apartment, because you can't pay rent if you don't have a job. And it's hard to get, let alone keep a job when doctor's appointments and excruciatingly debilitating pain take up most of your time, that you would normally spend working. I ended up staying at a relative's house in the next town over to finish my physical therapy and doctor's appointments that were linked to those two car accidents, and the subsequent legal cases. The same two car wrecks that led all my past injuries, from past accidents to the forefront of my life and physical health. My Mother and Grandmother had moved back to our small town that was once the embodiment of Andy Griffith's Mayberry. So, with no other choice, I too, eventually moved back home to Montrose, and back in with my mother and grandmother after I fulfilled my medical appointment obligations in relation to those two Colorado Springs car wrecks, and the court cases associated with them. If you think getting in a car wreck, or car wrecks, is a viable source of scammer's income, or a good way to get pain pills, let me not only point out that those accidents stay with you physically, but those were the only car accidents that I went to court over, and I was lucky to get $50,000. Unfortunately, it wasn't "take home" money. It happened to barely be enough to cover my incurred medical bills. In case you missed the point, I got bupkis, nothing, notta, zip, zilch, except a lifetime of chronic pain. The only silver lining, I was happy to not end up in medical bankruptcy. Sometimes, you have to take the wins you can get, even when they feel like a loss.

At my last appointment with him (you'll understand why it was my last with this doctor by the end of the next few paragraphs) Dr. Horedoor says, "Sometimes you can be on too many medications. And when that happens, they are actually making you feel worse than you are. They can exacerbate your existing conditions, which makes the experience of your symptoms seem way worse than they actually are or should be. Sort of an adverse reaction of taking too many medications."

I thought about what he had told me for a moment and replied, "Okay, great, you prescribed most of these medications for various ailments. My other few meds, from my other two providers, you are aware of and said you approved of, and you also believe them to be more beneficial than harmful. As have my other two providers in my case. So which ones do I stop by weaning off, and which ones can I just discontinue cold turkey?" I asked.

His exact response, and I'm not even kidding you, "I don't know."

"You can't help me anymore, can you?" I replied, looking back at him, my head halfcocked, kindly candy coating my disappointment, as it didn't seem like he had helped me at all.

"I don't think I can." He said. I could tell he was a little disappointed as well. Whether it was me, the situation, his performance, or the many limits of his occupation, etc. which one or ones, I had no idea. And at that point for me, that patient, all it meant was I was up a creek without a paddle. But I hadn't realized it yet. I also didn't know it was a sewage creek, but I figured that one out later too.

"Well cut me loose, I guess. And please refill all of my meds one last time, so I can get to the next medical provider. I'm going back home to Montrose. I've been told the medical field there has improved greatly, so I should be okay." Boy, did I end up being wrong. And like a person passing a hot potato, he was more than willing to quickly comply to get rid of me. So, I left almost as quickly as he dumped me.

False Hope Leading to Real Change

I moved back home, and at first, it felt good. After finding and seeing my new doctor, Dr. Feltheard, a few times and gauging him as a competent person and provider, I told him exactly what Dr. Horedoor told me. About how being over medicated can sometimes cause you to feel like you're doing worse than you really are. Dr. Feltheard looked at my list of medications and said, "Uh, I couldn't agree more. You are on way too many medications, especially for your age. Stop this one, this one, and this one," as he made check marks with his pen by the respective medications on my list. "And wean off of this one, this one, and this one," as he hand marked a "W" by those.

I did exactly as he told me. Weaned off these, immediately stopped those, and I can honestly say that I felt quite a bit of improvement after that. It was such a contrast that I thought I was more improved than I was. I would like to say that was the end of it and my further difficulties had nothing to do with being on way too many medications, for way too long, that lasted for far too many years, and it was solely due to the indelible mark that I left on my body by being in way too many accidents and injuries, but that was rather the tip of the iceberg of those related medication problems, as well as my future medical difficulties.

Were you paying attention? I said medication problems. As in legal government approved drugs did me more harm than good, most of the time, for most of my problems. Bad Doctor Dope is what I call any, and all, of those horrible and varied medications that gave me an experience that, in the recreational drug world, would've been referred to as a bad trip or a dirty/hot load, in best case scenarios. Where the medical field simply says, "adverse reactions." If they had any idea how horrible some, hell, most of those experiences can be, and were for me, they wouldn't be so nonchalant about over prescribing, let alone prescribing at all.

Speaking of which, is it ethical for someone to prescribe medications that can have severe, and sometimes, life altering consequences without those prescribers having experienced at least a simulation of a severe adverse reaction themselves? Because this is truly a realm where perspective is everything, and observation is akin to the Titanic spotting the infamous iceberg on the horizon and failing to immediately correct course from sheer hubris assumption of something like, "oh that's not so bad. We are in an unsinkable ship after all." For those who don't know that particular part of history, it ended very badly. Better to err on the side of caution. And most likely the origin of the saying, "that's only the tip of the iceberg." As the unforeseen danger often wreaks the most havoc. I also want to point out that most recreational drug users know to only buy drugs from a drug dealer who also takes the drugs they sell. The heroin, fentanyl, and meth dealers who don't do those drugs are the most financially successful for the longest time, but if the people who is selling it won't consume it…

Anyway, I was relieved to have found such a good doctor who listened. And I was also relieved to find out the rumors about the medical community improving in my small rural part of the state seemed to be true. But like the saying goes, "If it seems too good to be true, it probably is." And if it really is good, all good things must come to an end. Which is what I found out when Dr. Feltheard moved away for a career opportunity that would benefit his better half. This was shortly after he had a man-to-man conversation with me, encouraging me to apply for disability. As he put it, "you can't keep going like this, you have to apply for disability." And even though I, at first, fought him on it, I quickly realized that he was right, and I had no other choice.

But I, like a few of his other patients, were left to find another medical provider. Only I had the additional task of what Dr. Feltheard had tried to reason with me. The hard sell that I am disabled, and needed to be on disability, to a new provider who never even met me. Not looking as bad as you feel can be a blessing, unless you're trying to get help. Keeping in mind that not all disabilities are visible. This is when I began to realize that the positive rumors I heard about my small town catching up to modern-day standards with medical providers and facilities may have only been rumors after all, and highly exaggerated. And perhaps my faith in the medical field in general was overinflated.

It would also be less than a decade before government interference would once again level the playing field. But instead of making things better, which let's face it, politicians rarely do, they made it worse, for everyone across the board, patient and provider alike. Even though it downgraded everyone's healthcare, it downgraded healthcare for the people on the lower tiers with inferior insurance far less than it did for the people on the upper tiers with wealthy person insurance. So, when they said everyone deserves access to the same healthcare, who knew they meant eliminating the gap by knocking those on the top, down. Instead of elevating those on the bottom to a higher tier with better care. As that was how our leaders at the time were selling it.

Allow me to paint a picture of this current juncture of my life. My chronic pain was only in my neck, shoulders, upper, middle, and lower back. My pain was incredibly high, which caused pain-related insomnia. I had, and still have, undiagnosed events that may be neurological, maybe not, but most probably related to seizures, and yet not any type of seizures at all. Just seizure-like symptoms that let's say they make me fall down and spasm a bit as if I was actually having a seizure…but I'm still told that I'm not having seizures. And if that last sentence felt dizzying, imagine being the patient, thrown into the middle of that tornado of confusion by the medical field.

To top all of that off, most of the time, I couldn't even eat like a normal person, because if I wasn't nauseated, I was vomiting due to my typical twice a week migraine. By twice a week migraine, I mean I would have three days of a constant severe migraine, right into what I called a migraine hangover day. Which is where your migraine is gone, but that level of suffering was so intense and exhausting that you're wiped out, completely out of energy. And then I would dive right back into another three days of a consecutive, excruciating, horrendous migraine. On top of dealing with a new diagnosis of Delayed Onset Complex Post Traumatic Stress Disorder. That's when someone stuffs trauma deep down and hides it, until it finally builds enough pressure that it "pops the cork," as I like to say. A champagne bottle with too much pressure, that someone else decided to shake up until the inevitable conclusion. But it is really the emotional equivalent of a volcanic eruption. All thanks to an overzealous man who came to my door to try to intimidate me, as my father would have done, to someone who he viewed as a steppingstone, or an obstacle standing in his way. Triggering every mental trauma that I had managed to suppress up until that point (thanks again, Asshole). Which gave me even worse depression, because chronic pain, migraines, and an undiagnosed falling down and flopping around like a fish out of water syndrome wasn't depressing enough at twenty-eight, now anxiety attacks and severe depression plagued me. All thanks to the still unwelcome accomplice of my newest ailment at the time, P.T.S.D., and all the hell that comes with it.

Even after Dr. Feltheard helped to get me off a plethora of medications, I was still being prescribed, and taking, a wide variety of medications that seemed necessary, but would also turn out to be more harmful than helpful in my future. The prescriptions I was taking at that time were a pain killer, a muscle relaxer for obvious reasons, pain control and muscle spasm control, and I still take those two. They ended up being the only two prescriptions that helped more than they hurt me on a long-term basis. Plus, I had a new anxiety medication for my new anxiety attacks, a consolation prize that comes with all forms of PTSD. Who knew? A migraine abortion medication, for attempting to try and stop one of the most brutal experiences I have ever repeatedly had, and more times than I can count. A sleep aid, of course, to knock my broken ass out. Which worked less, and less, until they had the opposite effect that they were supposed to. A nausea medication because, well let's be honest, no one likes to puke, let alone feel like you're going to puke. Even our canine friends are so embarrassed about vomiting they immediately eat it, I'm convinced it is to hide it from us. A heartburn medication because the medications I've mentioned so far would eat a hole in anyone's gut. As well as a stool softener, medicated prescription numbing pads, and an initial therapy-only-no-more-drugs approach for my P.T.S.D. and depression. And also, my O.T.C. medications.

After repeatedly delving into my past traumas with my therapist and psychiatrist and deciding that hellish trial and error of head therapy didn't yield any noticeable results in a reasonable time frame, I gave in and opted to take antidepressants again. Antidepressants that had failed to help me previously. Antidepressants that my medical providers had repeatedly offered, and in some cases insisted, that I take again. "You're disabled. For that reason alone, you're depressed, and you need to take antidepressants." For making that decision, and taking that advice, I should've been committed (ironically, I eventually was). But I let them talk me into taking an antidepressant booster as well. No wonder I saw the inside of a mental stabilization unit! It is now very clear to me that when depression is situational, even if that situation is permanent like a disability, it is not a matter of correcting a chemical imbalance, and doing such is counter-productive in the long run. It is instead more imperative to learn to accept your current circumstances. After all, in a field that is merely "practicing medicine," do you really want them guessing what to add to your brain chemistry when brain chemistry to this day, isn't completely understood?

"Now you should feel content, even occasionally happy. But not too happy. Too happy means you are having an adverse reaction and even though it might feel really good, it is very bad as it will drop you further and harder later. You don't want that." Said Dr. Boyardi, who was my psychiatrist, when I finally broke down out of frustration at my lack of progress, gave in, and asked for the antidepressants that had been offered, and even pushed on me so many different times by so many different medical professionals.

"Understood. I'll try to watch for that." I replied. I can honestly say that I meant it. I've had to learn how to listen to my body through all of my medical trials, and I thought I had a better handle on it at that point than I did. Especially where an adverse reaction was concerned. In hindsight, it turns out that I have been depressed most, if not all of my life. What the hell did I know about what being too happy was?

No, at that time, the combination of Lexapro (an antidepressant) and Abilify (an antidepressant booster), all I knew was feeling way too good, felt really good, and it didn't feel excessively good either. My psychiatric medical providers even thought I was doing great and that I had turned a corner, what a major milestone! Even to the point of closing out my mental health case, as they thought I was doing that well.

Well, the Lexapro and Abilify combo really did make me feel way too good and I was enjoying it, probably way too much. It was like getting high without actually getting high. Somehow, I was getting high on life by cheating with something that isn't supposed to be intoxicating, just mood boosting. I was even smiling for no reason, and a lot. A grinning idiot who smiled and laughed at inappropriate times. Which, by the way, should've been another clue that I was having an adverse reaction. And while I was at the exact place that I was warned about without recognizing it, it really was so good, and I was loving it so much. We're talking barely under deliriously happy and if I'm being honest, at times beyond deliriously happy. If being high on life was actually like that, everyone would want it. Hell, maybe it is, and I don't know it. At that time, all I really knew was after being depressed for as long as I could remember, I now felt liberated.

To be happy, seemingly truly happy, even though it was artificial and entirely chemical, and had me way too elevated. Not to mention, it was the high point on a rollercoaster that would eventually drop me way too low and show me a new definition of pain and suffering. Not in a fun theme park roller-coaster way either. To be clear, that metaphor ends when you reach the apex. And to top that off I was still very much over-medicated and hadn't realized that yet either. So much so that with the antidepressants elevating me way too much as well, I was justifying taking a few drugs that weren't really helping me, without realizing that either. That's without realizing they weren't helping me, without realizing some were hurting me, and without realizing that I was justifying continued use. And who wouldn't? I wasn't taking anything that was illegal, and all I was trying to do was mitigate my various life altering ailments. Under the advice of my doctors who had no idea how high they were making me. And neither did I, until I came down. Who would've thought that medications that don't technically "get you high," that aren't on anybody's watchlist, and on nobody's radar, that are given to various patients like candy, would be the ones that caused some of the most damage, at least for me. Even though I can assure you I am not, and was not, alone in this thought or action. But does fault really lie solely with the patient? When was the last time you had a doctor explain what coming down from a high, or coming off of any medication, feels like to you? They should do this with all medications but antidepressants especially. Anytime someone is prescribed antidepressants they should be told that sooner or later they will let you down and at the least, an adjustment will need to be made. It could be a long and arduous process that could seemingly never level out.

"I'm an aspiring artist. I'm also a disabled man. Getting high and taking drugs is not only necessary, it's my prerogative." At least that's what I told myself and my friends during the time when I was first way over-medicated, starting at twenty-five years old and being prescribed thirteen different medications on top of my handful of over-the-counter meds. One of my ways of coping with that, more jokes, "I take more medications before five in the morning, than most senior citizens do all day." Dark humor has always been a good defense mechanism for me, and sometimes I can't help the play-on-words.

Around this time my anti-anxiety medication, 5 mg of Lorazepam (generic for Ativan and a minimal, reasonable dose), became the prevalent medication messing with me, and when I least needed it. I was taking care of life's little woes and not remembering I had done them. I procured a ride to Grand Junction, a town sixty miles away, to take care of some official personal business. A week or two later, not sure, I told that same someone who had already given me a ride, that I needed to go to Grand Junction so I could take care of that same business.

"We did that already, remember?" They said, concerningly. Of course I didn't. The generic Ativan was making me blackout, and I didn't even realize it, nor did I know how long I had been experiencing this adverse reaction to it. I also took my girlfriend to the hospital in an adjacent town, as she had a kidney stone that wouldn't pass. Apparently, I was a bit crass with the medical staff and even swerved in traffic on the highway during the drive back. I don't remember any of it. In my right frame of mind, and at that point in my life, I never would have driven in a condition where I had the potential to swerve in traffic. But blacked out on a generic benzodiazepine, all you need to do is ask, and apparently, I'm a Yes Man with zero recollection.

I was told another story about how I drove two of my closest friends around as their designated driver when they wanted to go out drinking one weekend. Because of my migraines I don't drink. For me, alcohol is a recipe for disaster (ironically, I've seen a much worse side of a few different medications, that are supposed to be safer than booze). It really takes the fun out of drinking alcohol when you can't even get to the end of a drink without it causing a migraine. It's like skipping the fun of the buzz, and even skipping being drunk as well, and diving right into the hangover, and that's sugar coating a severe migraine. But it also makes me the perfect designated driver.

In case you have never had one, a severe migraine is not like any hangover or bad headache that you may have and probably experienced before. If you have ever had a severe migraine, or have been close to anyone who has severe migraines, you know, or you should at least have a better idea, that it's so much worse than the worst hangover, or bad headache, that you have ever had (and I have had a few forty-eight hour long hangovers) and don't ask me which weekend that was either, I don't remember. Ha, just kidding, I remember them well, it's the six-eight hours following a swallowed benzodiazepine that I don't remember! As soon as I realized that I was, in fact, blacking out on my anxiety medication, I contacted my doctor's office and told them I was discontinuing it, and why. When you're not taking medication that makes you blackout anymore (a common occurrence with benzodiazepines, as well as what they have in common with alcohol, as they work on the same receptors), it starts to become much easier to notice other things that are happening and how your body feels. That's when I also started to notice other things about my other medications and remembering all of it.

After discontinuing my anxiety medications, I also noticed the need to discontinue my sleep aid medication. It started keeping me awake, rather than putting me to sleep. A common occurrence for anyone who is over prescribed sleep medications. Let's be clear, over-prescribed means I was told to take them every night for sleep, and I did, until that one no longer worked. Then I was switched to another one, until that one no longer knocked me out. And another and another until they all kept me awake. If you only take a sleep aid two-three nights a week, you'll likely not have this problem. As I should've been told but wasn't.

But seriously, before I had my migraines, I mostly misunderstood them. Firsthand experience can give a proper perspective. Before being personally struck down by severe migraines, I too was under the mistaken impression that they were little more than a really bad headache. This could not be more understated or misstated. It's as if you were to call having a sword thrust through your gut, that protruded all the way through your body and came out of your back, the equivalent of having a bad wooden splinter in your index finger. It really isn't a fair comparison. In a similar aspect, a severe migraine can feel like an icepick was jammed into your brain while that icepick magically and instantly grew sharp thorns and roots made of molten hot electricity, that painfully expands, penetrating ever deeper into your brain, with every excruciatingly throbbing painful intrusion, invading further in the deepest crevasses of your mind. While simultaneously, the thin layer of muscles that encases your skull spasms so tight it feels like an industrial hydraulic vise, squeezing your head inward from every angle, almost like an imploding star in slow motion. Only it is much more personal because you are experiencing the beginnings of that implosion while the stabbing electricity feeling inside of your head feels like it's still growing. Taking up more space than there is, rather than being an outside objectionable observer.

When I started having migraines at an exponential hyper speed and frequency more than most people do, my misunderstandings turned into brutal firsthand experiences. If someone didn't have the help from the medical field they needed when they had a severe migraine, they would be much more likely to do whatever they thought might help. Even if that help was life damaging or seen as notoriously nefarious. Whether someone experienced an occasional, rare, severe migraine, or what I did with three days of a single severe migraine, followed by a blessed day of unexpected and temporary reprieve that's more like coming out of a fog of pain into a unique pain-hangover, followed by another three solid days of head splitting, brain throbbing, stomach emptying, vomit inducing migraine, and the whole cycle repeated every week for years.

Almost everyone would try to self-medicate without proper medical support, but especially with the wrong medical support.

When my antidepressants eventually also did a 180 degree turn on me, dropping me like a ton of bricks, around four to six years after beginning them, or maybe that's when I noticed it. It was exactly like Dr. Boyardi warned me. "You want to be content, even happy on occasion, but not too happy, because if it makes you too happy, it will drop you further and harder down the road." He gives a slight dramatic pause with a serious stare when he summarizes with, "You don't want that." When they finally dropped me, it took almost two years to realize that my antidepressants had in fact dropped me so low, and so hard, that I couldn't even remember the last time I actually was happy, let alone content, and once again, it happened at the exact wrong time, because when else? I'm not sure what I expected, but in hindsight I really have been in and out of varying degrees of depression my whole life. Again, how would I have known what too happy was? But that's not all those two prescription medications did to me, or for me, for that matter, and in the spirit of remaining fair and objectionable, as being overly happy for a few years may not have been all bad, but the downfall after that sure was. When it did go bad, it was so bad that I couldn't even watch the five o'clock news without crying my eyes out, as if the travesties around the globe were happening to me personally. I'm not saying that world events aren't a matter of concern for everyone. I'm saying if you are that distraught over anything, you won't be able to do anything about it, even little things. It becomes counter-productive to lead any kind of life, except for one of constant despair.

Later I found out that a class action lawsuit was filed against Abilify, the antidepressant booster I was on. The lawsuit alleged that it could cause Obsessive Compulsive Behavior (OCD). It was especially noted in compulsive gambling and compulsive shopping, which was what the class action lawsuit focused on. I experienced a minor problem with gambling but I was highly constrained by the extreme limits of my meager budget, so I was never able to let it get out of hand enough to qualify for the class action lawsuit, as it was a minimum $10,000 loss, and that was more than I have ever had to lose or liquidate. I experienced a different side effect of Abilify in a more profound way. It made me obsessive about my pain and ailment management, while they simultaneously made all my medications not work, or made it seem like they didn't work.

When Lexapro and Abilify dropped me into a deeper pit of depression than I have ever been, they also seemed to encourage my other ailments to spiral out of control. As I mentioned, it made my other medications feel like they weren't working at all. Extreme emotional states would flip through my mind like the silver ball inside of a pinball machine. Being flung in an entirely different direction of thought by each bumper, flipper, or springboard. Each time the pinball contacted anything, it would trigger a different direction of thought of past betrayals and traumas, to another, and even another. I'd take a painkiller, and a muscle relaxer, and get nothing out of them. No pain or muscle spasm relief, not even a slight feeling of high to gauge if it was working. Smoke some medical marijuana, that always works…. Not under an adverse reaction of antidepressants apparently. The adverse reaction caused such a profound chemical block in my brain that at one point, I smoked almost all of the medical marijuana that I grew on my own for my first year, three pounds in three months. That is a quarter pound, a.k.a. four ounces, every week, all to myself. The little bit that I was able to share with other people absolutely obliterated them the way it should have. So, it's safe to say that it wasn't bunk weed, as my friends are no Green Horns.

While I was experiencing an adverse reaction to my antidepressant and antidepressant additive, I was also experiencing Serotonin Syndrome. Something else I had developed over the years, due to bad medication combinations, and way too many of them, for way too long. It was something else I had yet to be diagnosed with but would be down the road. It would also be caught too late for it to not be a permanent fixture on my chandelier of debilitating ailments. For those of you who don't know, Serotonin Syndrome is an adverse reaction to certain medications, and some specific medicinal herbs, that anyone can have. It is caused by the combination of certain medications. If the reaction is caught quickly enough, Serotonin Syndrome is temporary and fleeting. However, if a Serotonin Syndrome reaction isn't caught within a certain time frame, the Serotonin Syndrome can become long term and even permanent. I was given several of those bad prescription medication combinations. My medical providers not only didn't catch the severe Serotonin Syndrome reaction that I was having, but I also could have completely avoided it had my medical providers simply prescribed less. And it happened without any of them saying anything, until it was past the fact. And I have a sneaking suspicion through watching a few of my past cohorts and friends, it seems possible to cause Serotonin Syndrome with street drugs as well. But if I'm being honest, not being able to take certain medications and herbs is the least of bad things that will happen from prolonged use of the hardcore drugs, medications included. For example, it's horrible to take an anxiety medication to relax and have it black you out, like Ativan did to me. But it's even worse to take a single Xanax for the same reason, to relieve severe anxiety, and have it turn you into a rage monster. Just two separate adverse reactions that I have experienced out of many.

Funny thing about being generally over-medicated, setting the Serotonin Syndrome aside for a minute. For how many times being over-medicated happened to me, they all had a similar sensation, no matter the combinations. A feeling of being chemically separated from your environment. A feeling that I like to call Autopilot. The lights are on, and it looks like someone is home and at the helm, but it's more like a robot going through the motions of life. A feeling of chemical brain-fog that feels like you're experiencing life through a barely translucent veil, that translates to a feeling of being confused and out of place by chemical induction. As if looking through the veil of being over-medicated wasn't just a sensation that was only a hindrance to your sight, but a feeling that resonated the same way, threading through your mind and senses with a sort of white noise pain to it. Like having an ear exam, only the test tone is a constant uncomfortable feeling buzzing through your thoughts and mind, instead of a temporary sound cue in your ear, prompting you to raise your arm when you hear it.

When I finally realized that my antidepressants were not only no longer helping me, but in fact hurting me, I tried to think back to a good memory, to a happy moment. As long and hard as I thought, I couldn't even remember the last time I even felt content, let alone happy. So, I returned to the place that helped me the first time, our local mental health center. Only this time Dr. Boyardi had moved on, so I was placed with Dr. Snarls. His solution was this horrible mix and match trial and error with throwing various other antidepressants into the same chemical concoction that had left me mentally inept. Using at least one of the two culprits that started me down this path, over the course of eight months. The first thing that I explained to him was what Dr. Boyardi had warned me about, and how that exact event he had been so foreboding about had happened. I explained how Dr. Boyardi came to put me on 10 mg of Lexapro and 5 mg of Abilify, as Lexapro was the only antidepressant that sort of worked on a limited two-week basis, years before I saw Dr. Boyardi, and before the Delayed Onset PTSD came to the surface.

Dr. Ricki was my previous and first psychiatrist's name following the last two cat wrecks that changed my life. After his failings for a year and half with a plethora of different antidepressants in different classifications and only seeing minimal improvement of two weeks with minor benefits from one antidepressant called Lexapro, even though right after those two weeks of fleeting improvement, it immediately dropped me into one of my first chemically induced pits of depression. His logic was, "If it worked a little, on a fairly low dose, it should work longer and better on a higher dose." So, I went from 10 mg to 20 mg. Like the first time, for almost every antidepressant, it took four to six weeks to see if that dosage was working or not. "No? Still more depressed than you've ever been?" So, Dr. Ricki increased me from 20 mg to 40 mg daily. Another four to six weeks later, "Still not working for you? Well, you're in chronic pain and with chronic migraines. You're at maximum dosage so they are working for you, but you just don't realize it. Trust me, without the antidepressants you would feel even more depressed, so keep taking them."

Ironically, when I first moved back to Montrose, Lexapro was one of the first drugs that Dr. Feltheard told me to wean off, "If you're still very depressed then they are not helping you, no point in taking them." One of the first logical things that I had heard from a medical provider in a long time, and one of the few that I would ever hear. But he forgot to write it down in his notes. We're all human, after all.

At a later appointment, Feltheard also ended up being another doctor to tell me, "I didn't tell you to stop taking your antidepressants. You're disabled now. You need to take antidepressants." Just goes to show, doctors are flawed human beings too, with way too much on their plates. But at that point I realized his first assessment was correct. Why take any medication that doesn't help? Even if he didn't manage to record it or remember saying it. But again, this was before my P.T.S.D. was brought to the surface. Before I tried and felt like I failed to gain any ground with therapy alone after my P.T.S.D. was triggered. Before I caved and took the antidepressant Lexapro again, only this time adding the antidepressant booster, Abilify. It was before I had that incredibly strong adverse reaction to those two medications (and I use the term "medications" loosely) and before they dropped me like no other antidepressant, medication, or street drug had before, but not more than I would eventually experience.

Despite all of that, Dr. Snarls' ultimate solution to fixing my severe adverse reaction to Lexapro and Abilify…more drugs. Having already been through this specific trial and error before, I explained to Snarls the brutally hard time I had even finding an antidepressant that sort of worked, let alone one that didn't flip me out. When Snarls wouldn't bend to logic, I stated firmly, and with no uncertain circumstances, "Three times. I'll try three different times. If those three times are the same bad experiences that I have had before, when trying different antidepressants, I want to wean off and discontinue all antidepressants. If anything, for at least a short time period, so I can see where my head is at. Worst case scenario, I can start them again if things get too difficult. Best case scenario, I can start again from ground zero, with a clean slate."

"That's fair and I couldn't agree more." Dr. Snarls replied. I wouldn't find out until later that he was gaslighting me, and immediately before handing down his first set of instructions. "First understand that 10 mg of Lexapro and 5 mg of Abilify are very low dosages for those medications. I'm surprised you had any benefit at all." And right there should have been my first clue that what I told him about my previous antidepressant encounters went right in one ear and directly out the other. He went on to explain that he wanted me to increase my Lexapro to 20 mg from 10 mg and increase my Abilify to 10 mg from 5 mg daily. That was attempt number one. Who knew the medication that I was having a bad reaction to would give me a worse reaction with increased dosage? Huh. When it yielded more, and more depression and agitation over the next four to six weeks, and a lot more bad feelings, he knew that route was invalid.

His next attempt added 100 mg of Bupropion to my 20mg of Lexapro and 10 mg of Abilify combo that he wanted to leave me on. I'll hand it to him, adding the Bupropion did make me quit smoking, even if it was only temporary, but it was also because throwing that drug in the mix not only caused me to once again become suicidal, but it did so by causing what I have come to call "chemically induced apathy." Not, "I'm so high or so drunk that I don't care," apathy but rather "soul crushing, hollow-hearted, depression that makes you more apathetic than anyone should ever be," apathy. I didn't give a shit about anyone or anything, let alone smoking cigarettes. It wasn't a "hey, let's quit because I feel good, or want to feel good, or I had a moment of clarity, or even out of wanting to feel just a little better." I literally didn't even care enough to satisfy my addiction. It was more like "I deserve to go through nicotine withdrawals" and "I'm disabled, I don't deserve to feel anything at all." It was at that moment that I made the conscious decision that if I wasn't going to be able to feel anything, I should continue to smoke, just for an earlier death. When I reported exactly that was when Dr. Snarls decided that the Bupropion probably wasn't helping me and instructed me to discontinue it and lower my Abilify dosage back down to 5 mg and continue the Lexapro at 20 mg. That was attempt number two, in case you weren't paying attention. Four to six weeks later, and it was in fact closer to six, when I readjusted to not being on that combination, we tried something else.

At the end of those six weeks, I once again reiterated my original plan to him. If the next something else didn't work, I would be going to my plan that he, in the beginning, agreed was reasonable. If three tries equaled three fails, I would discontinue the antidepressants. Turned out that something else he had in mind, the third attempt, would be one of the most profoundly horrible drug-related experiences of my life, and one of my most painful and excruciating experiences as well. I still have side effects from it to this day. It was called Cymbalta. Dr. Snarls' instructions were as follows, and might I add, handwritten instructions that I still have.

They read…

-For 4 days decrease Lexapro to 10 mg a day, continue Abilify.

-Then stop Abilify, start Cymbalta 30 mg in Am, continue Lexapro 10mg in Am.

-In 2 weeks stop Lexapro, increase Cymbalta to 60 mg in Am.

For how incredibly uneasy I was regarding his plan, I decided I would try to plead with him to contact my old mental healthcare provider, and one of his former colleagues, at that mental health center, Dr. Boyardi. "I will not do that." Proudly proclaimed Dr. Snarls, at his patient's expense. I was blown away, dumbfounded, and distraught. This was clearly beyond his scope of capability, but he was too arrogant to put his patient's wellbeing and reasonable request first, which should be priority number one in any medical provider situation. Unfortunately, like any obedient, overly trusting patient who was more desperate than anything, I did as I was told. What choice did I have? I felt backed into a corner with no options but his, especially after he shut down my simple behest so quickly. It seemed, for him, it was a matter of if he reached out to a colleague, he would lose face because it would prove him incompetent in his field to one of his peers. Despite his obligation to put a patient's healthcare first.

Because of the difficult time I have had with antidepressants in the past, I asked two specific questions at that point. "When will I start to notice if Cymbalta will or won't work for me?" And "What do I do if I have another bad reaction?"

"Good questions." Snarls stated, with a look on his face that was both surprised and impressed. "Most people realize if Cymbalta will or won't work for them in four to ten days," Dr. Karls replied, telling me the only thing he said that didn't end up being total bullshit and in the worst way possible too! "If it does go sideways, discontinue the Cymbalta, and continue or restart the Lexapro and Abilify at your original dosage until I see you again but call and leave a message. Just to let me know."

"Ten days huh? That's a lot quicker than four to six weeks." I said, honestly a little relieved, stating the normal time frame for most antidepressants to do their thing was always a bit arduous when you're the one waiting and hoping for a positive outcome from a negative place. I agreed and promptly began the instructions given to me by Dr. Snarls, my psychiatrist, after seeing him on March 19th, 2015. Making March 20th, of course, day one. As instructed, I cut my Lexapro back down from 20 mg to 10 mg and continued my 5 mg of Abilify for four days. Each subsequent day, I felt a tiny incremental amount better. So already, I'm thinking this is going very well.

The next step was four days later. I discontinued the 5 mg of Abilify and started 30 mg of Cymbalta with my 10 mg of Lexapro. Keep in mind that Cymbalta won't kick in until after day four, but before day ten. And for the next four days, March 24th, 25th, 26th, 27th, I had the same tiny, yet noticeable, improvements that I experienced on the 20th, 21st, 22nd, and 23rd, when taking that first cutback step. Even on the morning of March 28th I still felt improvement. Until a bit later in the afternoon that day. Suddenly, the 28th went from still making tiny baby steps of noticeable progress, which is what you want, to complete mechanical failure, with an avalanche of anxiety flushing through my entire body and mind. Which is precisely what you don't want.

Still not fully realizing what had happened, I continued with Snarls' plan, that next day, the 29th. It's one of those ironic contrasts to taking an illegal drug to get high and having a very bad reaction, or a bad trip, versus taking a medication, or legal drug, to improve your health and having an adverse reaction. You almost expect it when it happens and you're taking an illegal drug to get high. It's one of those tacet caveats that everyone should understand and accept. Especially if you take hardcore street drugs, a bad experience can happen, and it very well might happen. You could get hurt. You could even die. But nobody expects a "bad trip" when taking legitimate medications legitimately. That being said, when medications do flip you out, it can take a minute to put what happened together. So that morning, the 29th, still flush with anxiety, I took 30 mg of Cymbalta and 10 mg of Lexapro, as I had the previous five days, as instructed per doctor's orders, and that day would prove to be one of the worst days in my life.

If that experience had been a small fraction less miserable, I may have been able to get off my couch, retrieve a gun, and end the exponential amount of suffering I was going through. And I wanted to, on that day, more than anything else, but I couldn't even move. As it was, the anguish and pain I was experiencing was so intense, it was paralyzing. All I could do was sit there in silence, and suffer in complete misery, like it took my voice away. It felt as if a black hole had opened inside of my chest. Like everything I ever was, and everything I ever would be, was being sucked inward, spiraling down into a black hole of oblivion, nestled deep where my heart used to be. And nobody would ever know what happened, not even the people sitting right next to me. My thoughts, memories, experiences, relationships, personality, knowledge, everything sucked in and crushed so small it became insignificant, unseen, and unrecoverable. That was when I realized it. I was having a bad reaction to the Cymbalta, and it wasn't going to work for me either. And even though I had the realization that my misery was in fact due to the Cymbalta, and it would most likely and eventually end, I still wanted it to end so badly, suicide was less than a slip of a lip away. But somehow, I managed to endure.

When I tried to go to sleep that same evening, I found a new gateway to this chemically induced hell whenever my legs would touch. For example, if my opposing ankles were to touch, or my knees, or my ankle on my left leg was to touch the calf of my right leg, or any other form of contact between my two opposing lower limbs, it would send these sensations throughout my legs that felt like a speed of light electric bolt being carved down my legs with charged razor blades. Now if you go to any doctor and describe a lightning bolt or electrical sensation, they think neuropathy, or some kind of nerve pain, but in this instance they'd be wrong. That feeling actually feels like electricity. What I was experiencing only followed that pattern but literally felt like it was being perpetrated and cut by razor blades and needles made of electricity and moving at lightning speed. I haven't been able to sleep with my legs touching since. Don't get me wrong, the sensation has changed and mellowed out in some ways over the years. Now, whenever my opposing left and right lower limbs touch, the locations that are touching instead feel like an incredibly heavy weight is pressing on wherever there are contacting locations. That sensation is also starting to dissipate…after a little more than a full decade.

It turned out there was also a class action lawsuit for exactly what Cymbalta did to me as well. The lawsuit alleged the pharmaceutical manufacturing company "fudged" their test results on how many people actually had a severe adverse reaction to it. The drug manufacturing company, during their own safety testing of their own medication (you heard that right, no oversight from outside of the company that was trying to create a new drug, investing in it, to trying to profit from it, was also responsible for testing it, to make sure it was safe, and self-reporting the results of those tests and studies). They claimed that out of the patients who took Cymbalta during the trial, only twelve percent experienced a severe adverse reaction. Which still seems like a high number to me, especially based on the intensity of the severe reactions from this medication, but again, I'm not a doctor. I'm one of the poor schmucks who was talked into taking it by a doctor. The lawsuit "alleged" that the percentage number of severe adverse reactions was modified, fudged, skewed, and the real percentage of people who experience a severe adverse reaction from Cymbalta was really fifty-two percent. But once again, I was disqualified from another lawsuit, unable to seek monetary compensation from something that hurt me for arbitrary reasons. This time, because anyone on poor person insurance only gets generic drugs. A few years before my awful experience with that specific medication, the Supreme Court ruled that generic drug companies could not be held accountable for the damage the drugs they manufacture do, as it is not their recipe.

I have some issues with that. First, generic drug companies are allowed to source cheaper ingredients in bulk, they are not subject to the same level of oversight, which has been inadequate to begin with, and mostly "self" regulated. As in the pharmaceutical companies, they have mainly been their own watchdogs. In addition, and perhaps more importantly, generic drugs only need a thirty percent absorption rate to achieve FDA approval. Whereas a brand name drug must have an eighty percent absorption rate to achieve FDA approval. Suggesting they must be different recipes, even though it is only "modified." Unfortunately when SCOTUS made that ruling, that generic drug companies could not be held accountable because it wasn't their recipe, they made a ruling that seemingly only affected poor and lower middle class Americans, which may be a bit biased in a nation that is supposed to do the most good for the most people, but I'm no lawyer either, or a one percenter. Furthermore, it seems if a company like Disney can now buy someone else's creative material and claim it as their intellectual property, even convincing some people (more and more everyday) that they even created it, and can thus now be held accountable for it, hence the censorship and editing in many films and shows, why is that so different for drug companies who manufacture other people's drugs? Another distinction without an actual difference. Except drug companies are killing people with these practices.

The next day I opted for my original plan with a "fuck this, Snarls has no clue as to what he is doing attitude," and discontinued the Cymbalta, continued my Lexapro 10 mg, and restarted my 5 mg of Abilify. I called our local mental health center and left a message with Snarls' pretentious assistant.

"Do you have Dr. Snarls' permission to discontinue your medications?" His assistant snidely asked. She was a very beautiful woman. Physically a ten in fact. But her shite attitude dropped her to a four, and that's being generous. Medical downfalls always suck, but it always makes it worse when you are in a bad way and you have to deal with bad attitudes.

"Oh, this is a courtesy call. I informed him what I would do if the Cymbalta also gave me an adverse reaction, which he said he was okay with as long as I let him know. Furthermore, it is unethical for you to try and dictate what I will or won't put in my body. As a medical professional, your job is to listen, diagnose, present options, and then do what the patient chooses. Anything beyond that and you are unethically exceeding your mandate. I will discuss this with Snarls at our next appointment." And I hung up. I may have been a little over sensitive as the Cymbalta still had me in a very bad place, but she and I never had a good rapport. After about two weeks of enduring the leftover horrors of Cymbalta, I was finally starting to feel like I was slowly slipping further away from that black hole feeling in my chest, and the Mount Vesuvius level of anxiety was dissipating enough that I knew it would eventually go away to at least a manageable level.

At my next appointment with Dr. Snarls, which was well past this event by more than a few weeks, I told him all the horrors I experienced being at the mercy of Cymbalta and summarized with, "I did what we agreed to if the Cymbalta messed with me and holy shit, did it ever. I returned to my original dosage of Lexapro and Abilify, but now, especially after that last experience, I would like to go with my original backup plan of weaning off and discontinuing my antidepressants. So, I can gauge my mental status for myself, unabated by foreign chemicals. Then, at the very least I can start at ground zero with different medications, again if, but especially if, things get really bad."

"You don't want to do that." Dr. Snarls firmly stated, going back on his word without one second of hesitation. What he said hit me so hard, he may as well have slapped me in the face.

"Yeah, pretty sure I do." I said, visibly frustrated at his clear betrayal. "Besides that, this was the plan. Remember? If the mix and match hell you put me through didn't work, and it didn't, that is what I would do. And that is what I want to do. You even agreed that was reasonable!" I exclaimed, becoming more, and more upset with being treated like an incompetent developmentally disabled child who can be lied to and manipulated, as if it was for my own good, rather than for his convenience.

"Yeah, I remember but, you still don't want to do that." Restated Dr. Snarls, this time it was bit firmer as if his condescending tone was eventually going to change my meager mind.

"Look, you've flipped me out three different times now, on three different horrible antidepressant combinations. You refuse to contact my last mental healthcare provider, Dr. Boyardi, despite his credentials and experience dwarfing your incompetence, I'm done. Tell me how to wean off them safely." I stated, just as firmly.

In a defiantly hateful tone he said, "Fine. Go home, cut your Lexapro in half and discontinue your Abilify, it's too small of a dose to matter anyway, in a week discontinue the other half a Lexapro."

I bluntly but cordially said, "Thank you for your time," as I walked out of his office and out of that mental health center forever. That was good-bye to bad rubbish. Arriving back home, ten minutes later, I had already decided that I would not only wean off my Lexapro at half the speed he advised, but I would cut my Abilify in half and wean off it first as well. I also decided I would take two weeks for each step instead of only one week. I asked my mother and one of my oldest and closest friends, if they would take shifts on suicide watch, in case I needed it, and turns out I did. Something else Dr. Snarls forgot to mention, but I'm sure it was "unintentional." Because if it was intentional, I surely have stake to at least a part of his soul.

Another reason I took the extra precautions of asking some people to be a lookout for me was because I was already brutally familiar with the nonchalant attitude some medical providers have for the severity of adverse reactions, as well as the total disregard for the unique chemical withdrawal symptoms each class of medications and individual drugs have, not just the addictive ones. Not to mention Dr. Snarls' obvious shortcomings within his own career and knowledge base. I'm glad I did too. After the Cymbalta, things were different, especially weaning off the Lexapro and Abilify combination, again. Which not only speaks volumes to a lack of understanding of these types of medications, Head meds, I call them. The SSRI, SNRIs, Tetracycline antidepressants, etc. Medical providers don't really know what they do in relation to brain chemistry, the indelible marks it leaves on your brain function, and the unforeseen effects it has on your normal psychology, or the interaction that happens between these different foreign chemicals when they are smuggled into your system, they meet and mix in the body and brain. It might sound like a fun party mixer, but it is not. There is also an almost complete lack of firsthand experience by medical professionals, and a necessity for both. Kind of like taser certification for law enforcement. They need to experience being tased before tasing someone else, and I'm only speaking on an ethical level. Medical providers should have to experience an adverse reaction at least once. I already know there are current medications that when combined cause temporary, yet severe, psychosis. Think of it like an educational ride through hell, and be grateful you get the temporary version, because for your patients that experience this, it may not be temporary. I believe it should be a part of being able to prescribe medications that can cause massively unbearable psychosis, extreme mental illness, as well as adverse physical reactions on their own, without being combined with any other drugs. The purpose of proper perspective is paramount for ethical perimeters. It would only need to be in a controlled constant observation environment and as I mentioned, with a combination of medications that have temporary, but also guaranteed, debilitating psychological side effects. Again, proper perspective is everything.

Weaning off Abilify and Lexapro the last time... What a bitch that was. I've had my fair share of accidents, injuries, surgeries, and illnesses, but this was another one of the worst experiences of my life. Especially on a mental breakdown level. I learned a sharp lesson on the relationship between one's physical and mental health. They are not only reliant on one another but also are dictated by each other. I call it The Teeter-Totter to Hell Theory. Imagine a flat plank like a long 2"x12" wooden board, commonly used for a teeter-totter on a playground for children. Only this plank doesn't sit on a fulcrum fixed a couple of feet above the ground. This metaphorical teeter-totter has no physical fulcrum. It is simply fixed to your baseline health as its fulcrum. On one end of the plank sits your physical health, where a child would normally sit on a playground teeter-totter. On the opposite end, where a similarly sized child would sit, opposite to where the first child sits, is where your mental health sits instead. When a patient has severe problems with both physical ailments and mental ailments, the two become tangible. A symbiont relationship. What affects one, affects the other, in a teeter-totter fashion. The difference is in the normal dynamics of when one child drops down, the other is raised up. With the Teeter-Totter to Hell when, for example, your physical ailments get worse, the physical side of course drops down. The mental side stays put at the same ground level as it and the physical side started at, where they were balanced. When your physical health worsened, the physical side of the teeter-totter dropped to a lower elevation, below the nominal normal healthy balanced lifeline. If the physical side stays down, eventually it will cause the mental side to drop. But not to an equal level of your physical status. Instead, it drops even lower, the same way the physical side first dropped. Now your physical side is still below the nominal level but higher than your mental side. Now your mental ailments' side is so much worse, hence lower than the physical side, now becoming the dominant ailments. The mental issues now outweigh the physical issues, even though the physical side is still as bad as it was, it becomes less noticeable, as your mental issues are now outweighing the physical ones. Taking the focus off the physical and putting it on the mental side. If the patient fails to elevate the mental side of their teeter-totter to at least a matching level of the physical side, the physical side will eventually, and again, drop further. To a level below where the mental side is at, once again the dominant pain/discomfort switching and the physical ailments become the more prevalent and more noticeable symptoms. If the physical side doesn't improve, once again it eventually drops the opposite mental side even lower again, once more switching which symptoms are more acute, while all physical and mental symptoms are constantly worsening. And it becomes a daunting descent into devastation.

I not only asked two people to be on suicide watch for me, while I weaned off and discontinued my antidepressant and antidepressant booster, but I asked two people that I cared deeply about. As I was more than aware of the deep psychological implications of watching someone die, or even simply witnessing blood and gore in real life. One of the many reasons I intentionally chose two people that I didn't want to hurt or harm in any way. And to expose someone to that, to leave your rotting or mangled corpse for someone you love to find, is cruel and only serves to perpetuate your own suffering, that you were trying to end. The sense of hypocrisy of that situation makes suicide an even more senseless act. In my life these two people were quite the opposite in fact. Two people I would do anything to protect and would never intentionally hurt. It served as another safety measure to be put in place.

When I was weaning off my antidepressants, I learned that the trick with the Teeter-Totter to Hell Theory, is to ascend each side as needed until both are back to a normal, or at least to an optimal and tolerable level. It is another way for a patient to monitor and gauge their own suffering. As well as gauge their own progress mitigating that suffering, while at the same time making them aware of that particular red flag.

For me, that meant fixing what was hindering any mental progress first, which at that time was my antidepressants. My precarious situation was so thick with irony I practically had to wade through it like sludge. Having too many medications prescribed, especially that can and did cause permanent and severe reactions to so many other medications, that now even a medication like an antidepressant, that should have made me less sad, now does the exact opposite. Like how a medication that should knock me out to help me get some sleep instead prevents me from sleeping and now keeps me awake. And how an anxiety relieving pill can make me uncharacteristically volatile and violent beyond measure instead of calming me down. Or even make me blackout, and I hadn't even figured all of that out yet. Not to mention the other brutal medication reactions that came before and after all of that.

When I considered all my past challenges with medications is when I decided to err on the side of caution and take a slower safer route off my head meds. It was no surprise that each of my two-week steps were pretty much an even more horrible sensation than any time before, and each time I gradually lessened my dosage. I compared it to falling backwards down a giant's ragged staircase, each step taking two weeks to tumble down, bouncing erratically off the chipped vertical cliff that formed walls, shelves, cracks, and crevasses between the broad flatness of the individual steps. Like rocks cascading down the face of a crumbling cliffside, or a stone silhouette like an old man's face cascading down the side of a mountain's edge, leaving a bare shapeless cliff (shout out to my New Hampshire peers, I know that one still stings). By the end of each of the two weeks, I felt like I was approaching more normalcy in the sense that I was headed in the correct direction, and I could tell it was going to get better. It would just take a long time as the progress, however noticeable, was also miniscule. At the beginning of each step came the kind of hesitation that sets in just before most people cliff dive, jump out of a plane, or bungee jump for the first time. It takes a certain kind of gumption to act against that natural, "you're going to die if you do this," instinct. Only no awesome adrenaline filled rush for a payoff. My payoff would come much later, as I slowly regained my sanity and presence of mind. That's when someone does roll call and you can stand up tall, with your hand raised and declare, "Here!" As opposed to being referred to as, "the lights are on, but nobody's home." It's similar for people who want to stop an addiction but don't want to go through the wretched sensations and feelings that it will take to stop that addiction. Or in my case, medications that were supposed to fix my depression that did the exact opposite.

Weaning off the Lexapro and Abilify post Cymbalta also came with a few extra unpleasant surprises. Every time my phone rang, I would have a panic attack. I ended up keeping my phone off for the majority of every day. I would turn it on once a day to check for messages, and that continued until I was far enough away from taking antidepressants that I was no longer having panic attacks with ringing phones. I also couldn't eat like a normal person. I wanted to, but I couldn't. It felt like I had to forcibly cram food down my throat, forcing myself to eat only to barely sustain enough energy for survival. A chemical induced anorexia. I also developed an aversion to eggs that made me nauseated if I smelled them being cooked. If I tried to eat them, they would make me vomit. Too bad too, I used to love scrambled egg sandwiches, and that is a symptom that persists to this day. Any form of citrus consumed, fruit or juice, started to make me sweat as if I was inside of a sweat lodge, sweating to the oldies. Except for the not working out part, I could've fooled Richard Simmons into thinking that I had been working out for hours. Citrus to this day still makes me sweat that much. I liked oranges too. Eating became such a problem that I dropped from one-hundred-forty pounds to one-hundred-fourteen pounds. At the beginning of each two-week-long-step that I incrementally lessened my dosage; I would start out as a sobbing emotional wreck from the act of weaning off and taking a lesser dose. Depriving my body and mind of medications that it became reliant on, to the end of the two weeks of torture, where my body would tell me I made the correct choice with the tiniest differences and improvements that were barely noticeable, but they were there.

I would love to tell you that after I weaned off and discontinued my antidepressant and antidepressant additive that I was, bing-bang-boom, all better, but it wasn't that cut and dry. It took a long time for Lexapro and Abilify to leave my system the rest of the way, years in fact, but I don't think it would've worked if that was the only thing I did. Like learning how to overcome an addiction includes more than stopping a drug, you also must learn how to live again. So did successfully getting off antidepressants and staying off them. While I was in the middle of my body and mind revolting from being cut off from a SSRI and additive, I noticed that any day that I didn't do something, especially contributing to running the household, I felt like a total bag of shit (honestly, rightfully so). It didn't matter that there were days when I didn't feel well enough to contribute. It didn't matter that I was and am legitimately disabled. When I at least helped a little, even if it hurt me and caused a pain flare-up, I at least gained a little self-worth and I would think to myself, "at least today you're not a total lazy ass shit bag, just mostly." Like I said, those "happy drugs" (antidepressants) eventually made me not-so-happy because of an adverse reaction that initially made me way too happy on them. When they did drop me, for years I didn't even feel worthy or deserving of living a decent life. That level of depression and despair makes it hard to clean your…well anything…dwelling and personal hygiene included. So one of the things I did along the way to accompany weaning off the antidepressants, which, keep in mind, didn't and couldn't become a daily thing until after I took that last two-week-step, as those steps were initially too debilitating, but after that I made myself do at least one chore every day, which I gradually increased. The self-worth was almost instant because even though I had to make myself do it, in the beginning, it was begrudgingly. Like I mentioned, I didn't feel like a total shit bag either, just mostly shitty. Finding motivation became easier and more rewarding as I slowly reminded myself what it felt like to actually work and earn my living. What it felt like to contribute and be a contributing member of society, or in this case, contributing to my household. Something else I did was make myself exercise. Well, in my case physical therapy, but again, good or bad physical health can help or hurt your mental health and vice versa. Like most things, it too started out slow and small. You do as much as you can without hurting yourself. Eventually you add more as you slightly improve and slowly make progress. It is slow, it is tedious, as well as arduous, but it is necessary. I also put my devices down. Brain rot is not only real, and slowly being recognized as such everywhere, but it is detrimental. Right now, the focus seems to only be on what it can do to a developing child's adolescent mind. But what does it do to an adult's mind? How about what does it do to an aging mind? The answer, about the same thing it does to an adolescent mind, fucks it up. It is the latest form of a drug that can be abused. It can do everything a drug can. It can make you dependent on it for an endorphin release, which can help brainwash you as there is no oversight, let alone laws in place for protecting people from it. It can even be more subtle than that, simply turning you complacent over time and slightly picking at your subconscious with subliminal messaging. It can make you slip your responsibilities. In any case, it is hard to make positive psychological progress when your conscious and subconscious are being constantly bombarded by negativity. Which is why I also started to question the validity of my social media accounts. I noticed a few things.

Leading up to my self-expulsion from social media's influence, I started to notice aberrant behavior. If I saw something I disagreed with, it was on. Suddenly, my fingers would float across the keyboard, stinging anything my keystrokes could reach. That was when I realized I was picking up any gauntlet I found, and none of them were thrown at me. I was putting myself through extra mental hardship, while I was trying to resolve the mental turmoil that had accumulated my whole life. It's much harder to put a fire out with gasoline and even more so when you are bathing in gas beforehand. Some might say it's impossible. And what I was doing was definitively counterproductive. Which led me to the conclusion that my social media accounts were in fact perpetuating my mental issues and I made the decision to delete my accounts.

What a relief it ended up being. Almost immediately my body and mind were able to take a sigh of relief. Even though I was one hundred percent resolved in my decision, I still noticed signs of an addiction. I kept reaching for my devices as if I was going to check my social media accounts and start doom scrolling. It was unconscious, like reaching for that cigarette after, well, after anything. As if an electronic device was just another addictive chemical. I can't even count how many times I would reach for one of my devices, stop myself by retracting my hand, while quickly clenching, releasing my fist by shaking my hand out to train myself to break that bad habit. I still, on occasion, catch myself doom scrolling through headlines and it always ends the same way, feeling like I wasted time, being sucked in and it usually puts me in a worse mood over things that I cannot and never could control. In my humble opinion, if you use your device more than a total of a few hours each day, there is no way it isn't affecting you adversely. The Chinese government apparently agrees with me, as they have set legal limits for their citizens. The European Union has also begun to pass laws that protect their citizens from the many harmful effects of electronic devices, and the shady business practices of tech companies that are becoming all too commonplace. American politicians have yet to even update a single law that prevents this or even regulates these companies for a little quality control. Slow down, do it right, and stop putting products out that are not ready for consumers, that are quickly antiquated, and that nefariously influence your customers. Everything about any smart device is made to be compulsive and obsessive, and hence detrimental to everything and everyone. Hence, a smart device is only smart for those who profit from it. For the rest of us they should be called dumb devices, because as convenient and handy as they are, they are making the rest of us dumber by the day. Seriously, when was the last time you had more than one or two phone numbers memorized that aren't yours? Or remember an important date or appointment without a reminder from your phone's calendar?

Another "side-effect" I discovered, post my electronic device addiction, was how profoundly bad being on my devices was on my body and posture. The whole, what is bad for the mind is bad for the body, and what is bad for the body, also bad for the mind. But it seems like an electronic device addiction is simultaneously bad for both mind and body. That leaves a multiplier on the Teeter-Totter to Hell Theory. A great example of this is the new sector of e-sports or also known as competitive gaming. If you notice, the teams and individuals that are successful for a long time typically find a balance between exercise and gaming to stay in peak performance.

If you are reading my book on an electronic device, I do apologize. It was my best course of action to reach the largest number of people. The greatest good for the greatest number of people possible. If you feel like my book is helping you, or may help you, or someone you know, as I obviously do (otherwise I wouldn't have written it), I encourage you to buy a printed copy, if it is available in your region. Keep it, loan it, give it, share it, help others with it, as I hope it will help you. Or at least take a screen break, set your phone or tablet down, and stretch your body, preferably outside to remind yourself there is a great big world out there. None of it is as good when viewed through someone else's lens.

So, let's recap a bit. Like everyone in the Eighties and Nineties (as well as before and after those decades) I was taught that all recreational drugs were bad, and all legal medications were good and mostly safe. Then I discovered some recreational drugs might not be as advertised by the powers that be. Finding out firsthand for myself (and loving it) and a lot of firsthand, that some recreational drugs, for the most part, were not what I, or what we, were told they were (WARNING: Some drugs will ruin your life by default. The other drugs can still ruin your life but like anything else, only if you let them). To being broke and homeless thanks to an almost century long prohibition on marijuana (and getting caught). Spending a year being homeless before cleaning my system out in two weeks so I could pass a urine analysis drug screening to get a job. And remaining sober and regaining the mental ground I held myself back from by indulging in recreational drugs at too young an age. Living and working totally sober and hence coherent, for my three plus years of being a tower hand, climbing, building, and repairing communication towers. As well as clean for most of the three plus years that followed as a medical office front desk receptionist. Until I was thrust into a medication induced walking coma with legitimately prescribed, albeit misunderstood medications, especially the chemical combinations, that I slowly brought myself out of with little more than a guiding hand from a few medical professionals, and at times, not even that much help, as well as the exact opposite. No help and even bad advice. So, I was left with mostly my own intuition and ability to listen to my own body that I have developed out of necessity.

Anytime I was overmedicated, it was a government sanctioned high that is the kind of high, and the level of a high, that most hardcore drug addicts would've been envious of. Only in reality, it delved me into years of hell with medications, alternative pain/ailment management, and at times a lack thereof. All to try to get better, but in that instance, under the influence of way too many medications, I was only able to obtain a pseudo quality of life. It was seemingly endless suffering, through a trial by fire of what helps more and what hurts more, until I finally found what gives me the best quality of life without unnecessarily sacrificing anything and at the same time being berated for it because the people who prescribe all of it, also misunderstand it. The whole, "it's a different story when you're in it," scenario. It is also psychology 101, when the shoe is on the other foot, it offers a completely different perspective. And despite conjecture of how you think you would handle it, it is almost always different when you are actually the one who is walking in those shoes.

And that is why you should listen to what I have to say. Because I was that person in that situation, I am that person who has learned how to handle it, and those are my shoes. That is why you should take the advice I'm giving. Because I survived, because I figured out how to maintain. Because I didn't let street drugs kill me, let alone control me. Because I broke my own desperate addiction to nicotine, and even though I only did meth four different times, I still felt that seemingly irresistible pull, from the very first time I tried it. It was something I was barely able to resist. I am very grateful that I was somehow able to resist it. And at the same time because of those types of experiences, I understand how easy it is to give in to that almost undeniable desire and how hard it is to turn it down. I also know if I had that experience with meth today, about thirty years later than I did, I most likely would not have fared so well. Methamphetamines are ten times as potent, and thus also more addictive now, as opposed to when I was an unruly teenager/pre-adult. You should also listen to me because I didn't let doctor prescribed medications turn me into an addict, kill me, or control me. And both street drugs and medication tried (whether on purpose or inadvertently). You should listen to me because I can keep you alive in these turbulent times or at least give you a better shot if you're going to cross that illicit line, or if you find yourself in a situation where you're reliant on medications, any medications. Or maybe you're a purveyor of medications or street drugs, and you could use or possibly need the proper perspective from the other side. It doesn't matter whether you are a recreational drug user, or a medication reliant medical patient, I'm speaking to you. It doesn't matter if you are a doctor, psychiatrist, pharmacist, medication manufacturer, cartel kingpin, street drug manufacturer, or a street dealer trying to make ends meet (because it's tough out there, I get it), I'm speaking to you. Because I can fill in the gaps and fix these problems if you will please take my advice. Enjoy longevity in life and in business. Don't, and it will end badly, whether it is your business or your life. Keep in mind there are many ways to live in poverty, but there are many more and worse ways for your life to end than death. And that's another last reason I'll give you as to why you should listen to me. I've lost friends because they thought they knew better. They thought they were somehow stronger than addiction, beyond overdosing, and above human psychology, but obviously, they weren't. As now they're either nearly hopelessly addicted, in prison, or dead.

So now you know. I am not just trying to teach you "how to do drugs," or "how to get high." Well, I am, but I'm trying to teach you "the best way to get high and not die," but really, it's "how to get high and lessen your risks," as well as "the safest way to take medications." Because people are going to take drugs for fun. People are going to need medications. And there will be more, and more medications that get put on the market and end up hurting more people than they help and possibly turn into the next newest street drug. Like it or not, there will always be new drugs, like Fentanyl. And there will always be people who overdo it and others who take advantage of that. My father comes to mind first and foremost, on a personal basis. The only guy I've ever known who could smoke four packs of premium cigarettes and wash them down with two eighteen packs of domestic beer, every day. Until he graduated to vodka because he thought people couldn't smell it. Guess what? Everyone can smell it, except the person drinking it. Vodka is about four nasal octaves short of ethanol. I'm also trying to teach you to pay attention to how your medications make you feel, your doctors are not empaths, there is no such thing (Shhh!).

And to the medical providers, moderation is key, and your patients are the best gauge for how well medications work. Listen to them, rather than the college educated salesman who works for the drug company and shmoozes you and your office staff with lattes from Starbucks and full lunches from Chilli's, Awesome Blossoms always included. A salesman is a salesman, as a narcotics dealer is a narcotics dealer, and the successful ones in both of those groups don't get high on their own supply, so how would they know what the drug, or drugs, they are pushing actually feels like or does? But a patient is the one who takes medication. So, listen to the people you're trying to serve and help, especially when they say the medication isn't helping, and even more so to those who tell you a medication is in fact hurting them, rather than those who are trying to help themselves by upselling you because their pay is commission based. Keep in mind, pain medications, especially opioid pain medications, are some of the best medications in your arsenal, and they go way further than you realize. To give everyone an herbal example, if Turmeric works well for relieving inflammation and discomfort in a certain patient, there is no immediate reason to put them on the concentrated version, Cumerin. Less is more. This is one of the methods you can use to responsibly prescribe narcotic painkillers, benzodiazepines, muscle relaxers, etc., without causing problems. Less is more.

Before, during, and after Nancy Reagan's D.A.R.E. program, drug education, especially in the 1980s, put out warnings everywhere. From the guy with the frying pan and the egg who fried it up on public service announcement commercials, the metaphorical drugs frying your brain, the egg being your brain, and the heated skillet being the drugs. "This is your brain," He said briefly holding up an egg, then cracking it on the side, dumping the egg's contents into a black cast iron skillet and setting it on the fire lit gas stovetop, as it instantly started to crackle from cooking, "This is your brain on drugs. Any questions?" If you were a smartass like my friends and I, then yeah, plenty, like "are you going to eat that?" Or "probably shouldn't crack your head open and spill your brains out, especially in a skillet. Unless you're Hannibal Lector." Or "you're doing drugs wrong!" There was the commercial, "No one ever says, I want to be a junkie when I grow up." As you see a guy who is clearly on drugs, and probably homeless, running down a street. As the camera zooms out, you realize he's being chased by the cops, and if you pictured a black guy, shame on you, it was a white dude (but caught you!). To the father (who was ethnic, not sure what the PR choice was there) yelling at his son. Demanding his son tell him who taught him how to do drugs. "Who taught you how to do this?" Until the kid snaps back at his father, returning the screams in both an offensive and defensive tone, "I learned it from watching you!" As the commercial flashes to a scene of his father smoking pot while being spied on through a keyhole, type of situation. All the way to the iconic "Just say No." Another pivotal world changing slogan from D.A.R.E. It might not have made much of a difference in the war on drugs, but it did make for a lot of great jokes, funny skits, and comedic routines.

I also want to point out that most parents who smoke marijuana end up doing so with their children. Some wait until their children are adults, but most take on a, "if they're doing it here at least they aren't out getting in trouble and doing worse" mentality. Whether that is a justification for ill behavior or a commonsense approach to handling something your children will indulge in anyway and thus viewing it as a way to keep things from getting too out-of-hand while also keeping your children and their friends as safe as possible, is a debate for people with children. My two cents are my friends that had parents that were "down," may have kept us from getting in more trouble than we did, or eventually did. Or perhaps it simply delayed the inevitable and only further held us back from growing up. Just some food for thought.

The Chicago Story, The Relevant Part

"You wanna know what hare-on's like?" He pauses and adds sternly, "I'll tell you what hare-on's like. Get in the next right turn lane."

Heroin was one of the few drugs you already knew you were being told the truth about how dangerous it is. Basically, don't fuck with heroin. Don't fuck with needles. Nonetheless, quite a few people get drawn into and hooked on heroin. And don't fool yourself into thinking one method of consumption is more or less addictive than another. Now there's fentanyl. If drugs were people, fentanyl would be heroin's bigger, badder, scarier cousin that got let off death row and out of prison on a technicality. And Car-fentanyl is his even worse twin brother. But if addictive substances, like and especially heroin and fentanyl are so harmful, so what is the draw? What's the appeal? Is the high from those drugs really so good it actually causes people to "chase the dragon?" It was certainly worth an inquiry. Especially since it has always been a curiosity of mine, even before I tried any recreational drugs. Morbid? Maybe a little. But if anyone could describe what heroin felt like, someone who had not only done heroin, but was hooked and honest about being hooked on it, surely, they could share that information. And I certainly wasn't inclined to cross that particular line myself, despite my curiosity, so a secondhand accounting never hurt anyone and was more than enough to satisfy this particular curiosity of mine.

It happened to be Puerto Rico's Constitution Day, 1998. My best friend Sonny and I were staying at a mutual friend's father's house in Joliet, Illinois for the weekend. Being young adults, and full of spit and vinegar, we decided to go into Chi-Town before heading to a college art summer program on Monday, put on by The Art Institute of Chicago. The Summer program was in a small tourist town in Michigan called Saugatuck. It was on the almost exact opposite side of Lake Michigan from Chicago. And no, you can't see Chicago from there or vice versa. The curvature of the earth won't allow it.

Did you hear that, Flat Earthers? THE CURVATURE OF THE EARTH. And I'm going to throw this out there. If you do drugs and you believe the earth is flat, it may be too late for you. Stop now. You may have done the wrong drugs the right way and had too much. Maybe you've had way too much of the right drugs the wrong way. Perhaps you took the wrong drugs or drug just once, in that case you may still have done too much, on a personal level or (and I'm joking here), but maybe you still haven't done enough, and maybe you didn't even need to do any at all. All joking aside, if you are this person, please stop now and get help. Doing drugs is no excuse for abhorrent behavior or thinking, and it needs to stop being an excuse. It's one of those things that perpetuates untrue stereotypes, makes it harder for us all, and keeps the perception of drugs in the dark ages of prohibition. And if you are a flat earther who has never done drugs and you still believe the world is flat, start.

When we headed into the heart of the thriving metropolis, we weren't only going to visit a big city and see the sights. We were headed to a well-known head shop to buy a new glass pipe in downtown Chicago, when we ran across a gentleman named D. There was nothing precocious about the way D looked. He didn't smell bad, he was far from belligerent or unruly, and he was every bit as clean cut as we were. Not at all what you would expect of a heroin addict. D was an African American of a similar age as us and wore similar clothing as we did. Sort of a laid back, post-grunge, stoner/skater style. If I'm being honest, I still prefer that style. Baggy, loose, and uber comfortable. D's hair was ultra curly, coal black, and a bit longer than mine was, at about shoulder length. We would quickly come to find out that he had a rather agreeable personality as well. The kind of guy you could hang with, have some good conversations on a regular basis, over a green bowl, or even the more popular and relatable barley and hops beverage, or perhaps a caffeinated beverage, or for those whose life or religion doesn't allow "additives," a conversation over a cup of tea and a card or board game, like Chess, or over a bowl of Life, while playing the game of Life.

Anyway, Sonny and I were walking up Such and Such Avenue when we came across D walking in the opposite direction. "Hey? You guys gotta lighter?" asked D. I normally would have assumed he asked us simply because of the similar garments. He saw us and knew we were "down," and for the same reasons we could tell right away, so was he. But I had watched him ask half a dozen people ahead of us for a lighter. Nonetheless, we could tell he was a partier. We, of course, weren't really sure what kind of "party" at that point, we simply knew he did. Turns out when he asked us for a lighter, he finally asked the right people.

"Hell yeah, man." Sonny immediately replied.

I added, "just a second…" as we both accommodatingly dug through our pockets. I found mine first, pulled it out of my left pocket, held it up, trying to spark it for him. Damned wind kept blowing it out. Still holding and flicking the lighter with my left, I cupped the top of my lighter with my right hand in an attempt to cushion the flame from the wrath of the nefarious Windy City. D leaned in sideways, also helping to cup the foreign flame from the wrath of the windy concrete paradise with his hands, all while trying to keep from burning his hair or eyebrows, and still getting his smoke lit, a smoker's curse. Sonny had moved upwind of us, and like a nicotine superhero, unzipped his jacket then he spread the opposing sides out like a bat, shrouding its prey with its wings, giving us a brief pause from the wind, as I was finally able to successfully spark a viable fire from my lighter. D inhaled sharply, pulling air through his cigarette, ensnaring the flame, with a quick deep breath, seducing the flame, finally engulfing the tip of his full-flavored generic cigarette, igniting a sustainable hot cherry of ember tobacco on the tip.

"Cool. Thanks man, nobody would lend me a lighter. I'm D." He said with the kind of relief in his voice that comes with satisfying a nicotine fit.

"You guys burn?" He asked, in a low tone code that only the three of us could hear, on that busy Chicago sidewalk, and he did it with a classic you-know-what's-up nod. Do you burn? Is one way to publicly ask someone if they smoke pot without being belligerent about it. Manners first, discretion always.

Obviously, our answer was yes. As such, we soon found ourselves back in my car, winding through the twisted and mixed cityscape that is Chicago with D now sitting shotgun, navigating for me, and Sonny sitting in the backseat, for security purposes.

"You mind if I shoot up?" D asked nonchalantly from my passenger seat as I drove through the busy streets of Chicago or some suburb thereof.

"Heroin?" I asked, as nonjudgmentally as I could possibly muster.

"Yeah. Most people I know…They won't even ask, they are such hardcore addicts they'll bang in front of anyone, anywhere. Even kids. Fucking crazy man. I'm not that bad. I think it's rude to not ask, know what I mean?"

"Huh, I appreciate that," I replied, acknowledging the need for decorum in any situation, but especially in the drug world. It keeps everyone safe. Similar to during World War II in Europe, when it was considered ill-mannered to have your hands under the table. Simply because it would make you suspect of being a spy. As I said, decorum keeps everyone safe, even now. "Absolutely, just do me a favor. Tell me what it feels like?"

"You wanna know what hare-on's like?" He pauses and adds a few lower octaves to his voice for a more serious tone, "I'll tell you what hare-on's like. Get in the next right turn lane." He takes a heavy breath and begins with, "don't ever do Hare-on." He said plain and sternly without any exclamation of anger, only emphasis.

I merge over to the next right turn lane in my 1997 Ford Escort as D continued. "I could give you an amount equal to the end of the tip of a pencil's worth and that's it. You're hooked for life. Your life is ruined." He stated firmly as he guided us through a labyrinth of streets beneath the cityscape's ground level. Driving directly through the devolved underbelly of Chicago, until we eventually popped out somewhere in the south side of the city. While we were driving through the underground gauntlet, he explained the areas on the sides of the underground roadways are fenced off to keep out homeless people, and addicts, and worse. "It doesn't matter though. They just climb over it or under it after a certain hour at night 'cause they know that no police are coming down here at night. Ya know, after a certain hour anyway." Finally emerging from the concrete canopy that is underneath Chicago, like coming out of a twisted mine at the base of concrete mountains, out onto a rundown city street that looked like someone dropped "ghetto" on top of Sesame Street.

"Park here." D said. We were maybe 50 yards from the underbelly of Chicago we emerged from as I pulled over, parking next to a dilapidated curb and sidewalk. He reaches his right hand into the right pocket of his big puffy baggy jacket. Taking another deep breath of satisfaction, an addict takes that's about to scratch that itch, simply a different addiction that he was about to "fix," as he simultaneously and slyly pulls out a small rolled up paper sack. He unrolls the wrinkled brown paper bag and begins to remove the contents. He continues with a stern tone, giving the dissertation of his life, "Seriously, don't ever do hare-on. It's the most…well…I don't know if…you know, if it's the worst...or not, but Hare-on is the most addictive drug in the world… yeah. There's nothing more addictive." He settles on, after verbally wrestling with the idea and deciding, it really was.

"I've never turned anyone onto it. No one. If anybody's on it, and they offer it to you, beat their asses, hard." He pauses for a second as he fiddles with his drug user's kit. "Seriously, that's fucked up. I never turned anyone on to it 'cause I know what it's like...Well I turned one person onto… but…like I've been doin' this shit since I was like Fifteen, ya know. He and I kinda started on it together…That person……." D briefly paused again, this time choking down some tears, "blew his brains out last year." He summarizes sullenly. Physically swallowing his grief, I could see his Adam's apple slide down and back up his throat, pushing his guilt back down, into the empty pit in his chest, where most men hide a majority of our grief. As he came back up, like emerging from the depths of an underwater cavern for air. He sat upright a little bit more, like a man does when owning his own mistakes and moving forward, and continued with his dissertation, "you have gotta maintain." Partially changing the subject with a minor redirection. He briefly pauses again while he begins to flatten out his brown paper sack by placing it in the hammocked lap of his baggy jeans, he starts rubbing the back of his right hand over the wrinkled paper sack, flattening it, while grasping the tools of his trade in his left and then methodically lines them all up. Setting them all out, lined up, on top of the now flattened brown lunch sack. Syringe, new needle, a metal bottle cap from a forty-ounce bottle of beer, a bottle of water, three tiny bags of dope dust, in this case heroin… "And you have got to be safe. I'm safe. Safe as anybody can be." He proclaims as he shakes each of his dope baggies, fondling each one, manipulating the granulated leftover scraps of drugs into his mickey's bottle cap, one bag at a time, until every molecule of heroin was gathered and accounted for. He adds a few drops of water from his water bottle into the mix.

"Here in Chicago, we got the Needle Exchange Program and the Green Card Program." He paused for a moment in silent concentration as he added a few more drops of water into the bottle cap from his fingertips. If he spills it here, there's no getting high, as he cautiously begins to heat it all from underneath the metal bottle cap. Melting the chunks of powdered heroin into the same cohesive liquid state as the water. All sitting together in the metal cap about to be fused together with my gas station brand lighter. As the concoction melted together, it looked like the kind of thing that comes out of your nose during a bad sinus infection, yellow, thick, and maybe even a little gelatinous. He held it with calloused fingers, immune from the heat after countless encounters with hot bottle caps and open lighter flames. "The needle exchange program. So, say I bring them one dirty needle, they give me ten clean ones. It cuts down on needle sharing and S.T.D.s. 'Cause fools be sharin' needles out here and getting A.I.D.S. and shit. I'm clean. I know 'cause I get tested at least twice a year. 'Cause you have got to be safe." He reiterated. "I never share a needle…well, I have, but it was like desperate times but like really desperate times, know what I'm sayin'?" He asked rhetorically, with a little chuckle. "I don't anymore though, too risky."

"Then there's the Green Card program. I'm an addict, on paper. Like, they have a record on me that says I'm a hare-on addict. So as long as I have my "Green Card," if the cops search me, they can't take my stuff, they can't take me to jail, nothin'. Not my shit, not my needles, not caps or spoons, nothin'. They know that people like me will just go get more as soon as we're out which just bogs the system down. So, it's kind of legal for us. They know if most of us can't afford it, we might break a law or two just to get it, so no sense in taking what we've already got. 'Cause you know, they think we're hopeless drug addicts who will never stop, 'cause it's that addictive. And mostly…they're right, man."

"I wrote a book 'cause well, I've been doin' hare-on since I was 15 and it's at my Momma's. Locked up in her safe. I'm gonna get it published… someday."

Securing the capped needle onto the plastic syringe, he unscrews the cap from the needle which seemed like to him, it was more akin to unsheathing a tiny hollow rapier from a tiny hard plastic sheath. A warrior always pulls their weapon with pride and anticipation of drawing blood, only a slightly different anticipation for an addict. He skillfully draws the liquified poison into the syringe from his metal bottle cap, filling a few CCs of the syringe as he pulls the plunger back. He fills another third of the syringe with water from the bottle of water he had. It's important to stay hydrated. He turns the syringe upright, pointing the needle straight up as if taunting God himself as he begins examining it. Neurotically, he begins tapping the syringe, methodically encouraging hundreds of tiny air bubbles to dance towards the top, away from the percussion of his fingernail rapping against the syringe's chamber, where all the air bubbles gather near the base of the needle in the plastic syringe. He compresses the needle to remove some of the air by quickly turning the needle and syringe downwards as he applies a small amount of pressure to the syringe's plunger. Purging the air and squirting a little liquid heroin onto the light beige carpet floor mat on the passenger side of my car and gently sets the loaded needle and syringe on his left thigh. Balancing it between the folds and waves of his baggy jeans.

As if he took another breath of grief and exhaled it in the same instant, this time with an almost heavenly sigh of relief. He continued again, as if his speech was unabated by another pause, "And when you're on "the shit" ya gotta keep your appearance up, that's the first thing to go, is your appearance. I bet you didn't even know I shot up." He stated, as he took his raggedy left shoe off. His white cotton sock, blood stained and stretched, we soon found out why, as with a hard and swift yank, he ripped it off his foot like a middle-aged man pulling the starter cord on his lawnmower after a long winter, yanking his sock clean off his foot in one swift jerk. With seemingly no time to spare he had it tied around his left bicep and cinched down with his right hand and teeth on the opposing side of the knot, the calf side of his sock, thank God! "Don't ever let anyone tell you that it's not a good high. Because hare-on's not only a good high, it's the greatest high, and I mean the best man." He excitedly announced with anticipation in his voice.

"That's why it'll get you hooked," as he snaps the fingers on his right hand, "like that, no problem, guaranteed. But you gotta be safe."

"Don't worry, I won't fall off on ya." D said with confidence as he finished prepping to shoot up.

"What's falling off?" Sonny asked from the back seat where he had been quietly and skeptically, observing and listening, this whole time.

"Falling off is when you just become worthless after shooting up. You can't conversate, you can't move, or hell, even defend yourself. You're just a puddle that used to be human 'til you come out of it anyway. Lots of fools get rolled because they fall off and somebody else takes advantage. Not me. I'm too seasoned." D bragged.

He slips the needle through the precipice of his skin, into his choice vein, on the inside of his left elbow. The one closest to me, in my car. He had it resting on my center console. He pulls back on the plunger, slowly drawing some blood into the mix of melted liquified heroin, unsterilized water, now also running a little red with his blood joining the mix inside the syringe. He lets go of the needle and it dangles from his vein. It hangs there like a marionette, retired at the end of a show while he sops up a wayward bloodstream slowly seeping from the side of the needle's intrusion in his dark brown and bruised skin. He barely managed to catch the blood drip with the wayward end of his tied off sock, right before it ran off the back side of his elbow. He plays with the needle a bit, moving it back and forth, to and fro, in and out, trying the plunger intermittently as it seemed stuck or plugged, then he let go of it again. Once more leaving it dangling from the inside of his elbow, like a partially attached appendage. I can both hear and feel my good friend cringe from the backseat. Not everyone does well with real life blood, and Sonny was one of them. D pulls the needle and syringe back out of his vein and clasps the end of his sock with the inside of his bent elbow to stop blood from squirting out of the freshly made hole. He held the needle upright again to loosen, or free up, whatever was holding the plunger back from dispensing his liquid fix. He taps it a few more times, shakes it vigorously, and proceeds to reinsert it, sliding it nearly back in the same vein hole, "Ah, there it is." He states with relief in his voice. An apparent yahtzee with finding his sweet spot, as this time he was able to slowly and steadily push the plunger down, forcing the semi-yellow, semi-clear liquid, now tainted pink with a splash of his blood, back into his vein, nestled in the crevasse of his elbow, on his left arm. The illicit concoction evacuated the plastic casing of the syringe and slid through the metal shaft of the needle into his vein like an alien snake made of liquid flesh, slithering into a mouse's den, like a well-planned and precision orchestrated invasion into an enemy's vital weak point.

It was almost like how the Grindhouse movies showed and pulp fiction books described it. As soon as he shot up, his eyes super dilated, his posture went from poor to jellyfish, almost appearing as if he had no spine, now barely more than a human puddle in my passenger seat. Suddenly, the car that was parked behind us turned their lights on.

D seemed startled by it, he slurred something that was practically inaudible, "Dri.."

"What?" I asked, hoping for a more audible answer.

"Drive." He managed to force out. At that point I was now certain the headlights freaked him out. I quickly complied, started my car, and drove the three of us away.

I asked D to describe what heroin was like. I meant what it felt like. Instead of telling us what I wanted and asked to hear, D told us what we needed to hear. He told us what it is like to live on heroin, to live with a hardcore addiction, and he also showed us. In retrospect, the whole experience was the most convincing, "do not do drugs" speech we would ever bear witness to and be a part of. I truly believe I was meant to convey this story. And if D hadn't fallen off, I can't even imagine how much worse that must be. As for the rest of the Chicago story, it will need to wait for another time, as for the purpose of this book, the most relevant part has concluded. As for the rest of this particular anecdote, I will simply say, to be continued another time.

Addiction and overindulging. They seemingly go together like love and marriage, or soup and sandwich. It's what we are trying to avoid, and at the same time we can use it as a red flag, a way to check yourself. Two of the ways a problem like addiction occurs, you can become addicted and begin to overindulge, or you can overindulge and become addicted. Essentially two paths to the same outcome, but keep in mind, not the only paths that lead to addiction. Unfortunately, some people are more susceptible to addiction than others, but in a world where more dangerous and more addictive drugs keep hitting the underground and pharmaceutical markets, there will come a time when the varying levels of susceptibility to addiction will be negligible and not matter at all, if that isn't the case already. As in, everyone who tries it gets hooked, no exceptions. And as D pointed out to us, in the case of heroin. But let me also explain by saying some people try drugs or alcohol and instantly that's all they want to do. And as much as possible, for the rest of their lives. I've always referred to it as having an addictive personality. In those instances, it is easier for some to make the justification to overindulge under the influence of addiction. To say to themselves, "I can endure any kind of hardship or degradation so long as I'm drunk/high." But it is a short-sighted plan.

There are also some who don't get addicted easily. Who can be weekend warriors and do recreational drugs occasionally. There are also people who can be given fentanyl, or morphine, in a hospital setting for surgery purposes, and never seek it out past that experience, where the drug was used for its intended purposes, in its intended way. One of the problems is, there's a limit. You can only do a highly addictive drug so many times before it hooks you, and I don't care who you are, no one is above addiction. In thinking that, "I'm a strong minded person," or "I'm above addiction," or "I'm too smart, or strong willed to let a substance control me." or anything else like that and you are deluding yourself when it comes to the hardcore drugs, and especially the newer hardcore drugs, but highly addictive drugs in general, medications included, just like my heroin addled Chicago acquaintance. That's when those people immediately or eventually become addicted. It's mainly by convincing themselves they are not susceptible. Unfortunately, no one is above human psychology. Especially where the inevitability of addiction is universal. In laymen's terms, fuck around on a long enough timeline, and sooner or later, you'll find out firsthand, a.k.a. the hard way.

Have you ever noticed someone overindulging in an activity? Can an activity be an addiction? Yes, absolutely. Take some known activities that are already considered problematic. Gambling, for example. In the case of gambling, people become addicted to the endorphin release that comes with winning, as well as the rush that comes with anticipation of a possible win. It can be an uplifting feeling when you not only tell yourself you're going to win but convince yourself of it. With excessive shopping, people get an endorphin release from not only getting something new, but also from the thrill of the hunt. But what about the not so obvious ones? Workaholics, for example? Ever seen someone with an addiction to electronic devices? Which brings us to some basic rules and guidelines. Not only for street drugs and medications, but also for life in general. I give you…

"The Golden Rules of Drug Use."

Rule One: Moderation

Moderation in all things, great and small. The moment moderation cannot be practiced; it becomes something that shouldn't be indulged in. That is when it becomes a problem. When it is life interrupting because of overindulgence. It is the surest sign of addiction. And addiction is what we are trying to avoid. Getting high without rolling the dice more than you have to because getting high can be dangerous enough. The moment putting it down, or going without, becomes difficult. The moment you feel that pull, that need, that desire, and it becomes a necessary part of life, when it is not. That is when you know you have a problem. Doing anything, but especially drugs, shouldn't interfere with your life. On any level. It therefore is important to find a balance. This means if you're doing drugs, you must always be able to "maintain moderation." If you don't do drugs, you should still learn to "maintain," as well. Maintaining means a few different things.

When someone maintains in life, they can indulge in life's little rewards, without taking any of them too far. And let's face it, there are many rewards in life. All of them can be taken too far, all of them can be abused. All of them can be harmful when overindulged in, one way or another. You can even overindulge in something most people do to get a reward, like work. But what if you could indulge yourself, without life's rewards indulging in you? Learn to maintain while high or intoxicated. Learn to maintain, in a conversation. Learn to take care of your responsibilities, first and foremost. You should be able to maintain a sober posture, physically. And let's be honest, good posture can help lead to good health. You need to learn to keep up, or even dominate in a game like chess, for example. People who maintain, also keep up with personal hygiene, maintain employment (because even if you're a dealer you gotta keep up appearances, but I'll get to that later), they maintain healthy relationships, and a healthy mental perspective.

I've heard it called selfcare recently, but personal hygiene and being healthy mentally are a necessary part of having a healthy life. Don't think because you do drugs doesn't mean you don't have to take care of yourself. No, it means there is extra selfcare if you want to stay under the radar, stay in the game, and not get taken down by what you are taking. A long time ago, it was laid out for my friend and I, by an older drug user who himself had been used by drugs, both before and again, long after he told us this. "One day this train ride has to end. If you don't choose to get off it, sooner or later, there are only two stops. Prison or an early death." And at one point, I really thought it might end up for me one of those two ways.

It is one of many experiences that led myself, and my group of friends, to adapt the recreational drug user's philosophy of, "you don't let a substance control you." We were convinced that with determination, sheer willpower, and true grit, we could achieve a perfect mind-over-matter state that would allow us to stave off not only all addictions, but most forms of brainwashing and subliminal messaging. What we didn't realize at the time is that it not only wasn't something that only the weak minded are susceptible to, but addiction is only a mind-over-matter situation to a certain point. When something is overindulged in, or something is so addictive it makes the strongest of people reliant on it, chemically or otherwise, it needs to be stopped and can be almost impossible for some to do so, hence the term "hooked." Like a fish caught by a fisherman, you're done. Especially for those notorious and hardcore substances that should never be indulged in by anyone. As the hardcore drugs are, more than likely, are something that will eventually take everyone and anyone who tries it. There may be people who handle it better than others, but sooner or later the hardcore drugs always handle you. Even the ones that are legal, including the ones that are medical.

This is where the education about drugs (recreational and prescription) needs to be concise, rather than labeling it all as the same level of bad. If you never lie, you're never caught in a lie. If you're caught in a lie, everything you said, or did, or will say or do, comes into question. Even the truth. This has a multiplier for businesses and organizations, and an even higher multiplier if it's from a government entity. This is where programs like D.A.R.E., that incorrectly teach, for example, that marijuana is an addictive, life ruining, gateway drug, and it will ruin your life in the exact same ways that fentanyl, amphetamines, cocaine, or heroin will. When people find out that marijuana isn't at all like what they were told, there is less hesitation in trying the other things you were warned about in the exact same doom and gloom way, that now seems far more likely to simply be more falsehoods. Even when they're not.

Let me try to rephrase that again. Marijuana has been labeled a "gateway drug" for a very long time. It is called this because it is believed, by outside observers, as in people who have never done drugs, that once you try marijuana it makes it easier, it makes you curious and even makes it inevitable that you will try more and even harder drugs. I believe this is a gross misconception. The real "gateway drug" is the miseducation itself.

"If they lied to me about something as minor as pot, who knows what else they lied to me about?" Is the thinking that leads down the troublesome path of hardcore drugs and life altering addictions. Not, "Well I tried getting stoned, I might as well chase the dragon now."

If you want to witness a visual representation of what the difference is in long term use, look at a picture of someone who has smoked pot all, most, or part of their lives. Compare that picture to someone who used crystal meth all, most, or part of their lives. A much shorter time frame, I know. But the contrast will be a person who looks completely normal and healthy, (well maybe a little overweight, but that's because the munchies are also a really fun part of smoking weed, or at least it can be!) versus a person in their late twenties or thirties who looks like a seventy or eighty-year-old, stage four cancer patient with partial, or no teeth. Essentially looking like a skeleton with unhealthy skin hanging down, off their bones. Would you really need to guess which one was the stoner?

If you are addicted…to anything, I'm so sorry. Please don't take my words as judgmental. No one really understands the unbelievable draw of an addiction, until you have personally dealt with one of those all-consuming sensations. And if you have been fortunate enough to have made it this far in life, and you haven't had the misfortune of experiencing an addiction, let me see if I can put it into perspective.

I think this is about the perfect example, because one of the things we were always told, and by told, I mean miseducated, is that the first one is always free. Well, your whole life breathing has been free. So, imagine if someone told you that you couldn't breathe anymore. Even more so, let's imagine someone, other than yourself, could actually make that decision for you and keep you from breathing, unless you pay for it. What happens? If not right away, very soon, you start to panic. Especially if you have nothing of value to pay with. Thoughts rapidly fire through your head. "I can't live without breathing! I'm going to die if you don't let me take a breath! How much do you want? Name your price! Just please let me breathe!" But you can't even speak to express all these thoughts without first being allowed to take a breath. Without being able to express your pleas, panic further ensues! An askew of biological, physiological, and psychological reactions put you into survival mode to fight, or scramble, or scam, or submit, or beg! Doing whatever you think you need to do to be able, hell, to be allowed to take a breath again! Maybe even kill, something you may have never really considered yourself capable of, until these horrible circumstances arose!

Now take it to the next level with your imagination. Picture taking that big deep breath of fresh clean air, filling the entirety of your lungs. It not only feels good and refreshing, as it normally does, but let's pretend it makes you feel really good, and for an extended period of time. Like, I won an Olympic gold medal event, good. Or I earned that coveted promotion that I've been working so hard for, good. Or I won the lottery, good feeling. It's one of the biggest appeals to doing drugs, alcohol included. The endorphin release, caused by imbibing something that makes you feel good, invincible, and even infallible.

Now, imagine someone again being able to prevent you from breathing, and once again doing it. Only this time they are also going to prevent you from having that really good feeling you got from breathing as well. And then telling you that you're going to feel horrible, for what seems like a long time, unless you pay them to let you breathe, and thus you will also get that great feeling again. Only this time that same breath that felt like heaven the first time wasn't going to be quite so wonderful. Still great, but not quite as good as that first breath. That will cost extra, because you'll need to breathe extra, and eventually that level will cost even more because you'll need more, and more, to get to that same or comparable level and avoid feeling horrible by coming down. It should take on a whole new meaning now. Sometimes it would be like, "I can't breathe, and I kind of want to just live, but if I can't have that really good feeling anymore, I'm not sure I want to breathe again, let alone live." And sometimes it's like, "I never want to feel that horrible coming down feeling again. I'll do whatever it takes to stay as high as possible for as long as possible and not come down." That is as close of a metaphor that I can give you as far as what an addiction to a hardcore drug feels like. It is a longing that will consume your soul and the need to satisfy it feels like a matter of survival. That is as much understanding and clarity as I can offer without that firsthand, hopelessly addicted experience. And I promise you don't want that experience. It is the draw, the pull of addictive drugs, hardcore addictive recreational street drugs, and addictive but can-be-useful-if-taken-correctly medical prescriptions.

I know what you're thinking, "I can't live without breathing, but I can absolutely live without drugs." Aside from a medical patient taking medication because they need to achieve a certain quality of life, or for furthering their longevity, aspects of drug use aside, and you'd be absolutely correct. However, with an addiction, that is similar to what it feels like when someone is desperately hooked. That is what it feels like when they run out, or have a hard time getting more, or are in a real-life situation where they must get clean, panic immediately ensues. It is the kind of panic that would normally only happen in one of life's actual harrowing situations. But "Oh my god, I'm going to die," is the one of the quintessential feelings of despair that an addict gets when they're faced with sobriety. Not only will they miss the high, but they also desperately don't want to come down and go through withdrawals. I was not so fortunate to escape my own demons unscathed. For me, nicotine was my fiercest nemesis.

Tobacco had its hooks in me so bad, so hardcore, that I had tried, and failed, to quit smoking so many times, even my friends, family, medical providers, and most of the time myself, never thought I'd be able to kick that habit. And how stupid is that addiction? Seriously, it gives you a mean head rush sensation for about thirty to sixty seconds, but only for the first half dozen cigarettes or so that you smoke. However, nothing that would constitute an actual "high," as you can achieve about the same sensation by impersonating The Whirling Dervish and spinning in a circle as fast and as long as you can, until you fall on your ass. And that's without getting the horrible taste of tobacco in your mouth, a rancid dirty smell on your clothing, skin, and hair, and eventually cancer, or a plethora of other medical conditions, and combinations of sicknesses and chronic health conditions, instead of only a bruise on your ass from getting too dizzy and falling down.

I call the smell of a tobacco smoker the scent of "Air Dirt." It's how a smoker smells after cigarette smoke has settled on your clothing, hair, and skin. The best way to describe it in one word would be grungy, but grungy to your nasal olfactory. Smokers can't smell it. Even though they reek of it. Only non-smokers can smell it. It's sort of similar to one of those, you are what you eat things, as current smokers can't smell it because their system, lives, and environment are saturated with it, making it a normal scent to them.

From beyond that initial beginner nicotine user point, after the first half dozen (give or take) cigarettes, or vapes, or dips, or snuffs that give you that head rush, you're only smoking to smoke. Vaping to vape. Dipping to dip. Snuffing to snuff. With any form of nicotine, there is no "high" after that initial short-lived sensation. You're literally maintaining an addiction with no benefit other than the promise of future health problems by satisfying a chemical addiction in your brain, all so you don't become irritable, even to the point of being a total dick, or a super bitch, like in most cases. People tell themselves it's good for stress relief and stressful situations, not realizing it is a chemical proprietor of anxiety and stress itself. Especially when you don't have it and can't get it right away. That's when the panic of a chemical addiction ensues.

When I finally managed to quit smoking, I didn't use one or two methods. I needed to use them all, a few tricks of my own, and the Governor of Colorado at the time even helped me out by making it harder to sustain my addiction. He made it way too expensive to continue to smoke by raising taxes so much they became unaffordable for my poor broke ass, especially brand name cigarettes. And even then, I still barely beat that demon. Speaks volumes to the lengths people will go through to satisfy an addiction, and how strong those addictions are, especially if you know how frugal I am. Frugality is necessary when you live on a budget, and yet, you still don't want to go without satisfying your addiction. I could barely afford my living expenses, and I couldn't always afford tobacco, but I still managed to feed the nicotine beast. Sometimes that meant picking up a stranger's cigarette butt. I know at least half of you gagged. Don't worry, I never lit a stranger's cigarette butt and smoked directly from it. You can pick up several sexually transmitted diseases that way. I would collect the butt, or butts, then empty the tobacco from them, discard the actual butt that was possibly contaminated with disease, wash my hands, then load the collected secondhand tobacco into a pipe and get my nic fix that way. Still disgusting, I know, but I wanted to demonstrate how desperate things can be when you have a brutal addiction and it feels like you have to scratch that itch, that is addiction.

I struggled with my brutal nicotine addiction for years. Over the course of damn near 2 decades, I tried and failed with this quit smoking method or that one, repeatedly. I failed more times than anyone should fail and still have the fortitude to keep trying. This last time I tried to quit, and finally succeeded, I used all the known quit smoking tricks, and a few of my own, as well, while taking advantage of current political affairs. In this instance, a sharp increase in taxes on cigarettes that shot the price of pre-rolled smokes in a box to the moon. My medicinal marijuana helped me a lot as well. If I had a nicotine craving that seemed like I wouldn't make it through I could smoke pot, for something to smoke, while simultaneously satisfying that oral fixation part of a cigarette addiction. I could smoke pot until I forgot that I wanted a cigarette, because my high would eventually outweigh my nicotine cravings. Or I would smoke until I needed to simply pass out and sleep through as many cravings as possible. And before you go there, I wasn't trading one addiction for another as get this, MARIJUANA IS NOT ADDICTIVE! I also let myself geek out on a roleplaying video game. I don't typically play those anymore because they can be life consuming. It goes against my whole "moderation in all things" theory. But for this one time, so I could accomplish my goals, I let myself get way too into one of them, one more time, for the sake of a distraction to help me quit smoking and I dominated. It wasn't really fair with my O.C.D. and pain-related insomnia, along with a desperate need for a distraction, most normal people couldn't keep up.

Otherwise, I also utilized some nicotine patches but very briefly, and way less than they recommend on the package. No sense in trading a smoking habit for a sticker habit. As well as many other distractions like hobbies, chores, and isolation when needed. I avoided mental triggers, gave myself rubber band snaps from a rubber band I wore around my wrist, not to punish myself for any reason, but to cause outside interference to my inner cravings, and I also tried to wear a fidget ring out. But again, my first biggest advantage to aid me in quitting smoking, admittedly, began when the votes came in to increase the tax on cigarette tobacco in Colorado in 2020. When that law took effect, I could no longer afford to be a Marlboro Man. So, I followed a good friend's lead and went to the local smoke shop and bought a bag of pipe tobacco and a box of what I call cigarette blanks, which are hollow cigarettes. Essentially, they are pre-filtered empty cigarettes without any tobacco in them yet, and I also purchased a cigarette rolling/packing machine. At that point, smoking cigarettes was affordable again, as long as I rolled my own. It was like having 1990's tobacco prices once more. Affordable, and it came with another unforeseen advantage.

Commercial cigarettes have so many chemicals in them, it is insane. Pipe tobacco doesn't. It is one of the reasons for the price difference. Pre-rolled cigarettes you buy in a pack use a wide variety of chemicals to make the tobacco last longer, taste better, burn slower, and yes, even be more addictive. Now, if you haven't put two and two together yet, let me point something out. Cigarettes were made more dangerous and more addictive by tobacco companies adding these varieties of chemicals. Instead of the government saying, "No, that's not okay for you to profit from destroying people's health," they pretty much said, "if you're going to use those dangerous chemicals at the expense of the people we are supposed to look out for, we will allow it, but only if you pay additional taxes on those chemicals." I'm adlibbing a little bit, but you get the picture. Shady drug dealers will do similar things. They will sell someone a highly addictive uncut substance for the first time, to get a long-term customer. The business transactions that follow, they sell a lesser quality, now cut product. Maximize supply to maximize profit at the expense of quality and the customer. Some will also give one of their customers a hot load to intentionally overdose them, only to promote their product. Or they lace certain drugs, like meth, with heroin, or fentanyl so that you get dope sick and then you feel like you have to come back. The main difference between big tobacco companies and drug dealers that will profit at your expense is….tricked you, there is no actual difference, save one is seen as shady illegal business practices that sometimes include murder, and attempted murder the other is condoned as business for profit by essentially paying a higher fee…yeah no actual difference. Whoever said for someone to succeed, someone else must lose, isn't on the short end of those death-sticks.

When I first switched to rolling my own cigarettes, two years before I was able to quit tobacco, I went through some initial, albeit comparably minor cigarette withdrawals from the lack of those various chemicals in my hand assembled nic sticks. It was similar to the withdrawals I have experienced over, and over, anytime I would try to quit smoking when I was smoking brand name cigarettes. But minor in comparison as I was only experiencing withdrawals from those added chemicals, not the actual nicotine/tobacco withdrawals. I truly believe that was one of the most important parts to my success in eventually quitting smoking tobacco, entirely successful this last time. A good friend of mine did the same thing. He switched to rolling his own around the same time I did, and we ended up quitting smoking tobacco at the same time together. He is of the same opinion about the chemical additives through his own experience of switching to self-rolled cigarettes and only then, years later, being able to successfully and finally kick the habit for good.

If you are actively battling an addiction, any addiction, don't give up the fight. Trust me, beating it can be done. You, more than most, know that draw, that pull, better than others and as daunting and irresistible as it seems, it can be resisted. It can be beaten. After you turn it down "X" amount of times, it gets easier to say no, walk away from, or even just be somewhere else. And, for your information, tobacco is not the only experience that I had with feeling the pull of addiction. It's simply the only one I had a definitive addiction problem with. For those fortunate enough to never have had an addiction, never felt that undeniable pull, hopefully now you have a greater perspective. If you have allowed yourself to.

Rule Two: Maintaining

First, patience is a virtue, and virtues are important. Not having patience is one of the first signs of addiction. As well as the first sign that you are failing to "maintain," rule number two. Which also means you need to check your "moderation," rule number one. If you go to a school event, work, or even a family gathering, and all you can think about is getting out of there so you can get high, or ducking around the corner so you can sneak a quick drink, take a pill, do a line, get a nic fix, or even take a hit, even feeling overly eager to get back to playing a video game, or compulsively check your social media in the middle of a visit or conversation, you, my friend, are developing, or have an addiction. Or, if you can't even get out of bed without the promise of a drink, or if you can't show up without being loaded, you have a problem. Unless, of course, you have a medical necessity. But, keep in mind, there is a difference between the desire for relief and the desire to satisfy an addict's itch.

Furthermore, when patience isn't practiced, stupid mistakes are made. People get caught because mistakes are made and sometimes people get hurt too. Relationships also get ruined because people get in a hurry and put too much priority on getting high and forget to take care of those you love. Because death can happen to anyone at any time, isn't a reason to seek it out. It is a reason to always be mindful of how we care for and treat ourselves, as well as others. Especially those who love us, and those who we in turn love.

You never know when the last time you see someone will be. Don't let it be a harsh memory or regret. As the saying goes, "Shit happens." So, try to watch where you step. Sometimes it's impossible to back track, depending on the size of the pile that you stepped in and the depths of the tread on your shoes. Hopefully you were wearing shoes. Nobody likes the feeling of fresh hot poo squeezing between your toes like playdoh coming out of a playdoh factory.

Know that having drugs is temporary and should be seen as such. You get drugs, to do drugs. Similar to how buying a six pack of beer or a bottle of booze should be. Either warrant a profound sense of moderation through self-control. Recreational substances are a brief escape from monotony and heartache, at best. Know that using a substance as an escape will not fix anything. It is only a temporary break and needs to be viewed as such. It is quite the opposite with overindulgence. Choose to do one of many hardcore drugs, or crawl into a bottle, and you will lose everything.

If you get drugs to sell drugs so you can make money, know that, for most, it is an almost never-ending downward spiral that only ends when you go to prison for a prolonged sentence, or when you die prematurely. Remember, the train ride eventually ends if you don't choose to get off, and the long and quick rides both begin when dealing with the wrong people. Keep in mind, dealing with the wrong people can also mean dealing with, and doing, the wrong drugs, as well as doing the wrong crimes. I don't condone crime as a way to get by, simply because it's shortsighted. But if you're going to be a criminal, don't be a hated criminal. Even most hardened criminals know there is a line, the smarter criminals do anyway. For example, drugs need to be done at an appropriate time and place. Again, it is a temporary break from stressors and reality. It should only be viewed as a temporary recreational experience. An artificial vacation from reality, but one you must come home from, otherwise you failed. It should be indulged in and viewed no differently than enjoying an alcoholic beverage responsibly. Doing drugs should only last as long as the high. Not after you've done the last of all your drugs you immediately get more. And innocents should never be involved.

That's one of the ways you know something shouldn't be indulged in. When people do it then they go get more. My friends and I used to call cocaine

"More" for that very reason. Get done doing a little, "Hey man, wanna do some More?"

Just finished the small amount of personal you and your buddy had, "Gotta go get some More."

An additional friend shows up, "Hang on, while I bust out a little More."

About to run out? "There's always More where that came from." And unfortunately, drug dealers, manufacturers, and distributors, a.k.a. organized criminal organizations know this, they exploit this, and they will continue to do this until users wise up, or a government finds a way to wipe them out. It's a losing business plan that only looks successful in the short term. It will come crashing down when enough people die, or are hurt, that you run out of clientele or it becomes counterproductive for world governments to let you continue. If you choose to get high on something that won't make you die, like weed, you never have those worries.

Know that you have to come down, and you need to come down, it is a part of the process, part of getting high, and you have to be okay with that. To put it another way, what goes up must come down. The current addict's mentality of getting more, to stay high is also shortsighted and needs to stop. It is essential to come down, so you can remain grounded in reality or so you can be re-grounded. Even for medical patients taking quality of life medications. A medication sabbatical, if possible (and it isn't always), can give perspective to a patient, as well as to the medical provider. Perspective as to where a patient's pain level actually is, and maybe even bring some masked ailments to the surface that were unintentionally being covered up. It can also give perspective to, if any, one's addiction level. If you fiend for the medication more than on a medical need, you might have or are developing an addiction. You need to be able to maintain and remain sober when you have to, and even more so, be sober more often than intoxicated, or at least more sober than intoxicated. So that you can handle life on life's terms. It is also a 100% better option to lower your tolerance level than to increase your dosage. I don't care what medication, or recreational substance, we're talking about. Less is more. If you increase the dosage exponentially until relief is found, the likelihood of causing additional problems, because you are unaware of your current problems, also increases exponentially as does the possibility of an overdose.

Simply put, the human body doesn't cope with, or like, foreign substances, but especially chemical ones.

When you begin to fight coming down, know you are starting to develop a problem. When you get high, ride the high, then come down. It is the total experience. If you get high and keep taking that drug to stay as high as possible, for as long as possible, that is when it is called abusing drugs. This also makes coming down much harsher. You have to take a pause for the cause, or more accurately, you must be able to take a break. This is the essence of maintaining. Especially when it comes to drug or alcohol use.

When I was first thrust into a situation where I needed long-term chronic pain management with potentially dangerous and addictive medications, they came with the same warnings, from almost every medical provider, as well as the same game plan. "When this medication doesn't work for your pain anymore, the only option is to increase your dosage. When that dosage doesn't work anymore, the only option is to increase your dosage or switch you to a stronger, more addictive medication. When that one doesn't work anymore, because of your tolerance, once again, the only option is to switch you to a stronger medication. Until you are eventually and hopelessly addicted." One of the major problems with this line of thinking is when someone does develop an addiction while taking prescription medications, it is typical to simply be cut-off by the medical provider and what they say is, "pain won't kill you." If the mental mentality is to cut a patient off when they develop an addiction only to tell the patient, the equivalent of "cowboy up." Wouldn't it be more logical to teach your patients to take occasional sabbaticals to offset their tolerance? Instead of causing a problem with over-prescribing with a never-ending increase followed by putting all of the responsibility on the patient. Or even better to learn to manage a medication on the lower levels of possible addiction, instead of exponentially increasing until the inevitable hardcore addiction? And even better than telling a patient to fuck off, they're on their own, which only to leads that patient into an addiction that begins by self-medicating with liquor or street drugs? Or even self-medicate as a better option than suicide? Pain won't kill you, sure. But try being in unmitigable pain and see how enticing ending it all seems after a certain amount of time.

This next part about "maintaining" is probably one of the most important aspects of it. People can suck. And I mean downright selfish, screwed up, greedy, take from you, before you can take from them, fucked up. Because they think if they'd do it to you, so will you do it to them. In that case, they might as well do it to you first. I'd like to think this is a small percentage of the population, but I've been wrong before. Perhaps it's only the percentage that thinks they won't get caught. So, if you're going to do drugs, you need to be able to protect yourself. Reading a situation and listening to that inner intuition that tells you to "get the fuck out." Perhaps it means you get in a bad situation, and help is but a loud yell away. Or you actually need to physically defend yourself from theft, assault, or the worst of crimes, sexual assault or murder.

It is impossible to maintain your own personal safety if you ignore moderation, and hence cannot maintain because you're so high, or so drunk, that you're essentially a helpless mannequin. If you do happen to become more intoxicated than you can bear (whether you took too much of a substance or were secretly dosed) and you can't "maintain," and something does happen to you, please understand what happened was still not your fault. People can be horrible, and whatever may have happened was on them. Your only fault was letting your guard down by becoming too intoxicated, by not maintaining. A hard lesson learned. If you were drugged without your knowledge, I'm so sorry you had that experience. It was a deprived individual(s) that took advantage of your situation, or you, and for their own selfish gains. What matters is how you move forward and what you do with that hard lesson and try to never let yourself be in that vulnerable position again. Keep your guard up by not getting too high, so to speak.

In life, you generally need to learn to maintain as well. And in all different types of relationships, situations, and various encounters. Empirical entanglements included and especially, if you walk the line. Encounters such as coming in contact with the law, or any other stressful, high intensity situation, it is very important to be able to maintain. Like running into any kind of authority figure. When I was young it meant parents and teachers, as well as law enforcement. But make no mistake, this is a different aspect of "maintaining." This is being able to handle a stressful situation, being able to "play it cool," as the saying goes. Or being able to handle an intense and stressful situation without falling apart but even taking charge and handling business in a respectable manner. Whether you're intoxicated or not, you need to know how to handle an emergency, as much as how to handle any situation that could be stressful, life changing, or even life ending. It's referred to as handling your shit. If you're in a stressful situation and you flip-out, you have failed to maintain, you failed to handle your shit (an ironic saying as some people actually get the shits when they get anxiety). But because you didn't handle your shit, you played the antagonist in your own story and thus made the situation worse (especially if you're one of those that get the shits!). Or, if you are so upset you go on a rant in front of law enforcement, or you're so stressed by the situation you can't even answer an officer's simple questions? Law enforcement, on every level, goes through training to catch someone in a lie, so if you're going to be a criminal, learn to lie better. Or an even smarter and better idea, don't lie at all. You can't catch someone in a lie if they're not lying! It's easier than it sounds. One tip, simply don't volunteer information, be polite and cordial, but not overly friendly.

If you're one of those people who are adamantly opposed to drugs, I'm sorry, but they aren't going anywhere. Time for a change in perception. And just in case it isn't clear at this point, another reason that you need to maintain, is so you don't develop an addiction. Do you like getting high? Of course you do! Drugs are fun! Similar to how drinking can be fun! Do you want to keep getting high and using drugs, or even keep drinking? Then maintain, and don't let a substance control you. But how? This is where you maintain (rule number two) again, with moderation (rule number one). When you know you've failed, is when your life changes for the worse, and yet the addictive substance(s) that helped get you there stays the same or becomes a more prevalent force in your life. Whether that's losing someone from your life because of probation, jail, prison, or impoverishment. Perhaps, and most likely, smaller losses leading to larger ones. Similar to an avalanche or rockslide that can begin with the smallest of antagonists. Maybe even leading to death, dismemberment, divorce, or becoming mentally deranged via chemical compounds. Honestly, most who overdo eventually become mentally incompetent by way of those chemical compounds, but I say potato-patato, a vegetable is a vegetable. You don't get to take your pick with those chances, but you can pick not to take those chances at all. With the hardcore drugs especially, it's not worth it. Plenty to get high on without risking it all to die. And you can choose not to overdo it with anything else in life as well. Finding balance is key for everyone with everything.

Rule Three: The Real Value of Drugs

Drugs are called dope for a reason. I would love to tell you that drugs don't have any value. The truth is most cost way more than they should, even though they don't really have tangible value. Medication should not be so overvalued either. I get it, everybody loves to make a profit, but if we all have prosperous health, we all profit far more, in far better, and many more various ways as well. Especially when you consider, from the drug dealer's perspective, any money earned from nefarious means can be questionable when spending it and can then lead to getting you busted. I believe anything that has the potential to ruin your life should be free, or close to it. From that same aspect, as well as the polar opposite, if medication not only has the potential to hurt you as well as the potential to help you, isn't that an even better reason why medications should be free? But the intoxicating delusion of dealing drugs, getting high for free, not working, and/or making a lot of money, can be tempting even though it is often a fleeting and shortsighted venture. Not to mention that someone who "hustles" for a living, instead of making a living working a job, will work longer hours, and ultimately will have nothing to show for it. Jimi Hendrix had a song about things like that. It's called "Castles Made of Sand." Illegal income is disposable income unless you break bigger and badder laws. So why even try drugs, let alone pay for them?

Once again, here's the harsh reality that no one who hasn't done drugs is going to like or understand. Drugs are really fucking fun…. until they aren't. They are incredibly enjoyable, and there is no experience like them, for better or worse. And that is why drugs cost, and can cost, a lot of money, because people are willing to pay for it. But when someone gets so high they don't even remember it, that's crossing one of those lines. You're either getting, or perpetuating, an addiction for only that, to keep the addiction going, no other reason. You wasted the money that you bought the drugs with. The drugs were a waste of your time and life because you don't even remember the experience. When you cross that line, or any line, with drugs, for drugs, to get drugs, or because of drugs, you have gone too far and most likely, you have done the wrong ones. Unfortunately, it is easy for anyone to do and makes it harder on all of us who don't abuse drugs or medications. Know if you do drugs, they should typically have very little or even no monetary value attached to them (and again, most shouldn't even have that).

In the underground world of recreational drugs everyone eventually gets ripped-off, taken advantage of, shorted, skunked. It is the ultimate test of how much value you actually put on drugs. Look, nobody likes being taken advantage of, and I have, in fact, been ripped off more times than I care to admit. And every time it is a giant slap in the face, and it will make you very upset, even angry. Here's how I have dealt with it. What if that little bit of coke or meth that you were rolled for, was the time that pushed you over the edge? That one time that took you from recreation drug user to full on addict. What if that was the dose that ended your life or sent you to prison? Consider it a bullet dodged. And if the person who dealt you a sour hand ends up getting in trouble or worse, you have abated a personal crisis at their expense, and it is their responsibility. Karma at its best. And I promise you, that when someone begins to steal, lie or cheat to get high, they will eventually cross that line, and probably already have. It leads to where no one should want to go.

When it comes to selling illegal drugs as income, know that you can always make more money and in better ways. Simply for the fact that ill-gotten gains may reap a large payday, but it is also disposable income. And if disposable income makes other people ask, "How'd this guy afford a boat and a BMW when he has no job?" At that point, you have been outed by your own hubris, vanity, and greed. The risk is not worth it, and sooner or later almost everyone who crosses that gets caught or worse. That being said, you don't sacrifice your friendships, or other relationships, to get it, do it, or make money off it. You don't steal to get it, you do not commit any act of violence to get it, and you don't allow yourself to have lustful thoughts of being high all the time. These are all examples of when doing drugs cost too much, and they are drugs you should personally not do, as you have put too much value on them, whether you realize it or not. And just in case you haven't noticed, you will struggle more, and hustle longer hours for money you might not be able to keep, than you otherwise would at a regular job with normal hours in a legal, way more versatile income. Keep in mind illicit money might and most likely will leave a paper trail that leads to your demise.

But what if it didn't have to be that way? What if you could get high and not let it ruin your life. Similar to some people who have a beer or two yet aren't alcoholics. It can be that way.

Also keep in mind that not all street drugs are purely recreational either. Some also have medicinal value. I'm sure you've heard the term "self-medicating." Well, like it or not, self-medicating with recreational drugs is a way some of us have survived trauma. Hardcore brutal trauma that typically only shows up on Lifetime movies for the mass majority of people. But if you have been paying attention to the real world, trauma is becoming much more commonplace now.

When drugs, the right drugs, that can be used with moderation, are used across the board in the same responsible manner as someone who has one drink or two (give or take) without being an alcoholic, is when doing drugs will begin to be seen as truly socially acceptable. Just as alcohol is. If some drugs that are recreational have an alternative medical purpose, and drugs that are medical by straight logic, also, and of course, have the potential for recreational use, there is also huge medical setbacks and side effects that aren't seen until they are released to the public, and then they are only seen with hindsight, what sense does it make to charge money for medication? Especially when the "long-term" testing is when it is released to the public. When it could improve the world or ruin it, but we'll never know which until we try, doesn't that run with its own similar risks as well? If medication was free, maybe there wouldn't be a rush to market for the sake of competition and profit. Pharmaceutical companies could go beyond the restraints of economic gains and instead see whose pill can help the most people. Maybe even work with one another for better results. Again, if we all have good health, humankind will prosper beyond comparison. There is no such thing as a miracle drug…but shouldn't there be? One with no side effects that cures what it is intended to, instead of only offering regimented treatment?

Harmful medications have the potential to do similarly harmful things as hardcore street drugs do and sometimes, even worse. They give temporary relief, even false hope, and then they show you hell by giving you worse side effects than the ailments you were trying to alleviate. All the things you never wanted. A healthy population is a productive population. An unhealthy population is only trying to survive by any means necessary. One of the many things I have learned since becoming and being disabled. When life is miserable, life can be one day at a time, and sometimes only an hour at a time. Medication can help that. Medication can also make that worse. Medical professionals should all say, "Less is more." The conscientious ones do anyway.

When medication that provides a better quality of life fails, or becomes unavailable for any number of reasons, one of a few things is likely to happen. Hopefully, the individual realizes they are doing better without it, and they begin to thrive. Or they realize how invaluable their medication is, and they have the harsh realization that life only gets so good and it is because of the medication(s) but then they can start to accept and come to terms with that. In the case of medications that have the potential to be addictive, sometimes a person simply doesn't get over wanting that high, even if they don't need the medical benefits of the medications anymore, so they look for it and for similar things through illicit means. A similar problem can begin by self-medicating with highly addictive drugs when the medications an individual truly needs becomes unavailable. Which typically leads to worse addictions and ends with prison, or abrupt and premature death, that is otherwise avoidable. Or an individual who doesn't want to cross that line and risk becoming a junkie or hardcore addict only to realize how essential those medications are to their quality of life, addictive or not, so they suffer, and suffer, and suffer. Until they decide they have suffered long enough and too much. That is when a patient can cross another illicit line. Whether with street drugs, counterfeit drugs, lead pills, gravity bombs, or other means, they self-medicate by taking their own life. If you've ever experienced an exponential amount of suffering, especially for an extended period of time, for months, or even years, and maybe you still are, I'm willing to bet that you know exactly what I'm talking about. It's easy to lose hope when it feels like the medical professionals that should be helping you don't care. I'm not saying all medical providers don't care, I believe most of them do. But right now, there's more than a few wrenches gumming up the gears. Hopefully this book helps to fix some or all of it.

You have a three-pronged problem that has spawned a tsunami of other issues. One is a lack of perspective. No other person can feel what you're feeling, what you're experiencing, not even a medical provider. Not on a physical level or a mental level, but especially where pain is concerned. You may have some shared trauma with someone, but I promise you that no matter how similar the shared experience was and is, pain and suffering is still vastly different for each, and every person.

Second, there seems to be an epidemic of negative thought among the majority of healthcare providers. It is a change in mentality that I have noticed from older medical providers to newer medical providers. Newer medical providers do less exams, with more conversations, while at the same time having two go to answers. One, the patient is always lying. Stop imitating entertainment, especially House. The patient didn't come into your office to lie. They came to you for help. When you assume they are lying, you fail to listen. The other answer is a shoulder shrug, which leads to the third problem.

Any professional who gets paid a premium for showing up, whether they do or don't get the job done, and still gets paid, has very little motivation to actually complete the job, especially the challenging ones. Or at the very least, less motivation than the rest of us have in our various careers. It's a lack of work ethic and a direct result from excuses like, "that's why they call it practicing medicine." Know that a work ethic is more than showing up and putting in long hours. It is also completing the job and doing it well. If you don't get the job done every time, you fail to have an actual work ethic, and in that case, you only have a work effort. When someone gets paid by default, it takes away any motivation to go the extra mile, or sometimes even negates the professionals' need to get the job done at all. When someone gets paid no matter what, why take on something that could be challenging? Why not earn the easy money? Which has led to my favorite, and all too common, blow-off line by medical professionals, "let's wait and see." The most expensive shoulder shrug you will ever hear. So much for being proactive about your health. I promise you, when medical professionals start getting paid after their patient is better, and not before, the medical field gets fixed, really quick. Forcing them to put their big brains together and come up with a solution so they still get paid, and we the patients all get fixed, instead of only helping a select few.

For those who haven't experienced physical or mental suffering and anguish on a severe level and extended basis, and thus haven't needed medical support for long periods of time, let alone permanently, you need to know when the FDA and CDC declared a national emergency on opioids, it was really only because of two pain medications that never should've been invented, let alone released to the public. There was a slew of medical professionals, and in Veterans Affairs especially, that took that opportunity to cut off as many patients and veterans as possible from these and similar medications. Medications that helped at least enough to make life livable for a lot of people. When they took as many people off a variety of pain killing medications as possible, "in the patient's best interest," despite the protest of the patients' which was mistaken for addict talk, a very large problem was caused. And don't get me wrong, I'm not saying there wasn't an element of addiction in at least some of the cases. I'm saying when someone hurts so bad they are completely miserable, it makes death start looking desirable. Who gives a fuck about possible addiction? Especially when it comes to having quality of life or not, but even more so for our veterans who have sacrificed everything so we can have a better life. It is a complete dereliction of duty when our nation fails our soldiers in any way, but especially when we let them down in a medical way.

The idea is to achieve quality of life. Suicide is the complete lack of and end to life. Thus, the worst quality of life one can have. What followed when our government overreacted, and overreached, was a ton of people, especially veterans, who decided that if the V.A., or the medical field, wasn't going to help them, and in some cases were making things worse with "alternative" and "off-label" pain medications, then they would end their suffering the only real way to end suffering. As human beings we owe everyone common decency, but especially our veterans, whom we owe much more than that. Imagine how bad they felt when they realized their sacrifices and suffering didn't seem to matter to the nation and people they served.

The thinking is, "If I have suffered a lot without medication, versus suffering a little with medication, and I can no longer have the quality of life that my medication provided, that would at least make things bearable, then I'll just eat a bullet and not suffer anymore." For those without religious beliefs, this isn't such a bad proposition. The lights simply go out. No Heaven, no Hell. Friedrich Nietzsche's endgame. That would also mean no more life experiences, or anything for that matter, because it is over. When there is that much pain, that much mental discord, that much suffering, it is easy to feel like you have nothing to lose. whether you have religious beliefs or not.

For those within the confines of most religious beliefs, it is an unthinkable act to take one's own life, or any life for that matter, until an inordinate amount of suffering makes you lose faith and take the ultimate gamble. Lose faith in doctors, in God, in humanity, and in yourself. Because if a medical professional, who, by definition, is supposed to care, will let you suffer needlessly, simply because he, or she, doesn't have proper perspective. Lacking that firsthand perspective because if they had it, they would be a patient instead of a medical provider, with similar or worse complaints. In that place, there always seems to be less evidence of God's existence, as well as humanity's worth. When there are justifications like, "We don't want you getting high on your medications." So, they give you no medications at all, or medications they think should work, but often don't in the capacity a patient needs or may even have some unintended consequences. If someone is disabled, or worse, dying, getting a little high every once in a while, is a good thing. And in the extreme of unfortunate medical circumstances, it isn't necessarily a bad thing either.

Sorry to be the one to inform the medical field and burst your bubble, but that misconception was warping your perspective like a fisheye lens on a camera. The intoxication part of many medications allows for a tiny bit of enjoyment, where it otherwise is a seemingly empty and dark void full of never-ending pain, discomfort, and depression. Laughter and joy are medicine, and a positive attitude is paramount when overcoming or learning to cope with any kind of sickness, disease, or injury. We have known that for a long time now. But when you're so miserable you don't even smile, you're incredibly grumpy and irritable, and you hurt so bad that life sucks beyond what it ever has before, it's almost essential to counter that with a short period of artificial chemically induced happiness and that can sometimes be absolutely necessary to break the cycle of a pain flare-up. As far as ending one's own suffering, I'm more of a Pascal's Wager kind of guy. It states, and a bit more elegantly than this, that "an intelligent man would believe in God as he has nothing to lose if he's wrong, and everything to gain if he's right." That being said, I can't count how many times my physical or mental issues have taken me to that point. Where suicide seems more merciful than being self-malicious by simply continuing to exist. In those moments the only real question is, "Would God understand?"

So, how many more lives have to be lost before the medical field realizes how invaluable opioid medications are? And yeah, I get it, so do most people, that medical professionals don't want people getting high because you think patients will start taking it only to get high, and they will continue to want to get higher, and higher, both taking and needing more, and stronger, medications, abusing it until eventual overdosing. But again, it doesn't have to be that way.

What if I again told you part of the problem was in the education? Only in this instance, the miseducation is about when and how to prescribe these and other medications, and what these medications do and feel like to the individual taking them. Medications that have incredible medical potential, but get misused because of their minor, yet profound similarities with street drugs. And yes, some street drugs started being seen as, and created as, viable medications, like heroin and cocaine around one hundred years ago. Except for heroin and cocaine and fentanyl, the problem is not the medications themselves. The problem, as I have been saying, is in the education about opioids and other potentially addictive medications as well as the lack of personal perspective from firsthand experiences. A patient who has never done drugs or had any kind of firsthand experience with addiction or addictive substances, or even no experience with intoxicating substances, cannot be expected to be able to handle it. It's the equivalent of being thrown into the lion's den, bound and gagged. You're simply not going to make it out unscathed, if you make it out at all. Someone who has never done drugs, also cannot teach you how to handle them. They're guessing at best. It's one of those situations where some smart assed medical professional would say, "That's why they call it practicing medicine." You honestly shouldn't make a top earning career salary if you're only practicing. Even professional athletes don't really get paid millions of dollars to practice. They get paid inordinate amounts of money to perform. They practice to improve and hone their craft and skills so they can continue to make more money than anyone should.

As I mentioned, being taught how to control, let alone how to watch yourself for addiction, is a task that would be almost impossible for someone who has never done drugs or had an addiction. And an equally impossible task for some who had an out-of-control addiction, as their experience was, or is, an uncontrollable one. That is one of my many goals here. To teach control with what is misunderstood but can be more beneficial than harmful. So that we don't continue to see more damage caused without these lifesaving medications. And eliminate the damage caused by abusing drugs. It also points out one of the problems with drawing a hardline between calling street and recreational drugs all inclusively dangerous and prescription medications as kosher, or even acceptably safe. Drugs are drugs. I don't care if you get them from the corner pusher or the corner pharmacy…use all with caution.

A doctor, or medical professional, who has no or limited experience with using recreational substances, let alone with addictive substances, also can't possibly competently teach someone about addiction and what to look out for. Especially someone who is just starting to take medication that has the potential for abuse, because again, medical professionals have typically never had that experience themselves. The experience of learning how to "handle it." But I have, and I'm going to tell you how to teach your patients how to handle their medications. And how the patients can watch themselves as they will not only need to, but you, as a medical provider, need to make it clear that if they ignore the warning signs and develop a serious addiction, it is on them, entirely. Because these medications are too valuable, and too useful to put blame on the medication itself, or the medical provider, except for cases of extreme abuse, like prescription pad happy pill mill providers. I'm going to teach you how to check your patients for addiction without crossing the constitutional line of innocent until proven guilty. Because giving someone drug screenings, by default, is crossing that exact line. In this country it is innocent until proven guilty, not assumed and preemptive guilt. I'm going to tell you how to show your patients that their pain medications are still blocking pain after their personal tolerance takes away most of the "high" part. And how, at that point, it is still exponentially more helpful with pain than a handful of Tylenol (Note: do not take a handful of Tylenol, it very well could kill you). And I'm going to show everyone how to "handle it" themselves, as you might be using, or on something harmful and addictive right now and you don't even realize it.

Remember, no matter how much drugs do or don't cost, cash is king. Everybody loves cash, and you should too! You should never use debit cards or credit cards. It leaves an electronic footprint. You should never write someone a check for drugs. Bad idea, it leaves a written record of it, complete with a copy of your handwriting and signature. It is the equivalent of handing the police a signed, handwritten confession, like robbing a bank but leaving a signed I Owe You. Drugs should never be bought on a front either. For those of you unfamiliar with the term "a front," think of it as buy now, pay later. As people who do drugs can be forgetful and unreliable because they let themselves become that way, as do the many varieties of people they deal with, and let's face it, shit happens, like it or not. So, cash upfront only, to avoid additional and unforeseen problems. This is where people get killed and commit violence for a deal gone bad. It's not so much that it was a drug deal that went bad and ended in violence but rather a business deal where one party feels they got the short end and was so upset by it, they retaliate with violence. It should be an unacceptable, taboo response. As should screwing someone else over so you can profit. But plenty of people have acted and reacted this exact same way, with no drugs or criminal activity being involved at all, and unfortunately people still do. Somebody felt cheated, was treated poorly, or one party got greedy. That same somebody took it too far and retaliated/acted out, in violence. The golden rule states, "treat others how you would like to be treated," works both ways. You treat someone poorly, it can come back on you, things can get dark, maybe even violent. If it is cash up front, it takes this problem off the table. At least when dealing with, "the illicit." This gives you another reason to keep a job. If you have the money, there's no need to buy drugs on credit, or to try to steal to get your drugs. If you do, it means you are lusting for drugs. Like trying to find a passive "get high" income, which is breaking the second rule. And you also need to remember D.A.R.E. Not Nancy Reagan's D.A.R.E. which is Drug Abuse Resistance Education, but the grounded in reality acronym of D.A.R.E., Drugs Are Really Expensive. In more than a few ways.

Rule Four: No Warning Signs for Addiction

Know, that because something is illegal doesn't mean it is dangerous, and even more so, it doesn't mean that it isn't dangerous. If it is legal and still dangerous on the same levels as hardcore street drugs, you may never know it, until it's too late. If it's not dangerous and still illegal, it's misunderstood.

In 1998 I turned eighteen. I was first in line at the DMV that morning, dressed semi-decently with a fancy hairdo, as I had more of it then, all so I could look my best for an unwinnable, non-re-doable, over eighteen driver's license picture, and not to mention an eagerness for the day. After being handed a warm freshly printed and laminated new driver's license that said I was officially an adult, I headed to the post office to fill out my due diligence. Every American boy's rite of passage into manhood, The Draft Registration. It was never completely lost on me, the cost of freedom, nor the freedoms I had already been afforded that others elsewhere around the world have not. As well as the many service members, and their sacrifices, that made those freedoms possible. I understood it as much as someone could who hadn't served their country. Nor was it lost on me, the liberties I had already taken and might take in the future. That would probably earn me a life sentence or two in a communist or socialist country, possibly including, but not limited to, writing this book. And the many men and women who sacrificed their health, and even their lives for.

Now our government has decided to sign up young men almost automatically. This should be a mandatory intentional act performed as a duty, not the same process as signing up for a free website or social media account. It should be something that you go do yourself, in person, and it should be done with heavy relevance and reflection. It is a reality check that freedom isn't free and one day you may be called on to defend these liberties and freedoms you have indulged in and enjoyed for so long, as many before have to obtain and keep our prosperous way of life. If you are called on, how will you answer? Will you help to extend those liberties and freedoms to future generations?

After that, all important civil duty had been taken care of, I drove directly to one of our local convenience stores. In 1998, in Colorado, if you were eighteen years old or older, it was legal to purchase, possess, and use different forms of gambling, like lottery tickets and lottery scratchers, as well as pornography, and tobacco.

"Hello," I said with a giant shit eating grin on my face, to a tiny Hispanic woman in her fifties, behind the counter at one of our local, raggedy small town gas stations. "I would like a pack of cigarettes, a one-dollar lottery scratcher, and a copy of Hustler magazine, please."

"Got identification!" She sharply exclaimed in a harsh tone, without even the courtesy of having her eyebrows raised in suspicion. Her stone-cold poker face indicated she was dead certain that she was about to catch someone underage trying to buy some things he shouldn't even have in the first place.

"Yes ma'am." I proudly and respectfully replied as I handed her my shiny new driver's license.

She takes it, and while she inspects it, I see her look go from a skeptical cold poker face to raising both eyebrows, in a "oh wow, he is legit," thought, that was reflected by her facial expression relaxing as she hands my identification back to me and almost apologetically said, "Happy birthday." As she begins to gather and ring up my requests of behind-the-counter, over-eighteen-only products.

"Thank you." I replied, still grinning ear to ear, as I paid for my gains and headed out the door.

How I usually tell this story is, "when I turned eighteen, I bought a lotto ticket, a porn mag., and a pack of smokes, and I'll be damned if smoking wasn't the only habit that stuck."

When I told that story, that way, at a quit smoking class put on by the state of Colorado's Health and Human Services, the lady who was running the class said, "That is by far, the funniest starting to smoke stories that I have ever heard." And as funny as that story was, the draw, the pull, that comes with being addicted to cigarettes was horrendous and has been proven to be one of the biggest banes in my life. An addiction, a serious addiction, is a longing that consumes you. One of my hardest, most brutal obstacles, and at the same time, probably one of my greatest personal victories when I finally managed to quit after more than a decade and half of failed attempts. When I did finally manage to quit, what I learned is, may God help those who are addicted to something worse, like alcohol, meth, heroin, fentanyl, and many different prescription medications. At the same time, I'm not sure you can call any addiction worse than any other. They all put an iron grip hold on the people who have become reliant on this addiction or that one. There is a difference with what a socially tolerated addiction does to a person long term, versus what a socially unacceptable addiction does to a person long term. Hence the socially unacceptable part. The difference is bad versus worse, potentially dangerous versus absolutely detrimental.

Considering that, it seems everyone either misuses or misunderstands drugs. The younger the generation, the further they take it. And it has now been taken way too far. Now, far too many have died. And even though medical providers write prescriptions, they misunderstand drugs so much. That they are now afraid of one of the most useful classes of medications they have at their disposal, opioids. And of course they are. People who have never done them, medically or recreationally, have the wrong impression because of prohibition, misinformation, and misrepresentation. Learn about something all you want, a firsthand accounting is always a different, more clairvoyant perspective. I have had a rather unique experience of being taught and raised to be adamantly opposed to drugs. Then having my eyes opened to drugs, out of curiosity. Eventually doing them recreationally, and perhaps also inadvertently self-medicating with recreational drugs, until it left myself and my first roommate, through no fault of his, evicted and homeless in our early adulthood, because of the ongoing prohibition of marijuana at the time and my own unwillingness to follow the law by indulging in something I personally felt should've been legal all along. To stopping recreational drugs all together (yes, alcohol and eventually tobacco included), staying sober, and gaining the mental ground that I had held myself back from by being a curious, wild, and unruly teenager. Only to wind up a ward of the medical field, back on drugs, once again. Only this time legally sanctioned dope, written by legally sanctioned medical providers, a.k.a. doctors, and becoming reliant on the two, the drugs and the doctors, for quality-of-life. Let me tell you, there is a huge contrast between doing drugs for fun and taking drugs that are labeled medication, just to be able to function halfway normally. It literally takes most, if not all of the fun out of it. But I can also honestly say that without my specific, unique experience experimenting with various drugs as a wild teen and crazy young adult, I wouldn't have survived what the medical field put me through, let alone survived what they gave me. At least Alice had the white rabbit to guide her. I wouldn't have known how, without what I already saw and experienced. I not only wouldn't have been able to recognize what the medical field tried to do to me (hopefully inadvertently, unintentionally, and solely due to the ignorance that often accompanies hubris) and thus I wouldn't have been able to stop it before it went too far. No wonder so many have needlessly died or became addicted. Especially since the most dangerous drug adverse reactions that I experienced weren't from street drugs, or even medications that are on anyone's radar for being potentially dangerous. As in, nobody is talking about the real monsters in the medicine closet. Without my specific experience and knowledge, it's almost unavoidable to develop issues that you don't want. When I think of what it would take for a medical professional to have my perspective…they wouldn't be medical professionals. At that point, they'd be patients. Like me, maybe like yourself, or someone you know or love. They wouldn't have had the opportunity to gain a higher education. They would've only been more wards of the medical field instead of being the stewards. They would more than likely end up being additional victims of the shortcomings of the medical field, more over medicated, and addicted than getting better. Simply because they wouldn't know what to watch out for.

That is why I decided that it's up to me to bridge the gap. It's up to me to straighten out the misconceptions and hopefully save lives. Because after all, there's no reason we can't all get a little high and not die. Especially in a day and age when we are starting to look at what was seen as no more than street drugs, are now getting a second chance as medicine. So here it is. Where everyone who has gone wrong, went wrong, and who helped it go wrong, and didn't even realize it. Here is how to check yourself for addiction, for every person.

First, how do you know if you have or are about to fuck up? I don't mean "ow, I stubbed my toe." or "I didn't bring my vehicle to a stop soon enough, so I rear ended the vehicle in front of me." Not to belittle how devastating a car wreck can be, even a minor one. A lot of energy and energy distribution in something with as much weight and inertia as car wrecks. But still no. I'm afraid this is a life-altering and even life-ending, fuck up. If you take any drug, recreational or medical, and you start to fiend for it, it is a craving. Not to be mistaken for the mouthwatering craving that you get when someone, or something, reminds you of one of your favorite chocolate souffles, or your favorite bubblegum ice cream from that old fashioned creamery in that now tourist trap of a mountain town. A craving on a fiend level is an almost irresistible pull that eventually turns into an almost impossible temptation to turn down. Especially after you have given in to that draw, that pull, so many times. Sometimes it's only once, sometimes it's a couple, and sometimes it takes more than a few. The fish that continues to nibble will eventually get hooked.

You'll start out with an anxiety-like feeling, mixed with anticipation meets overeagerness. Know that you shouldn't have anxiety about doing anything. This anxiety comes from knowing you're about to do something you shouldn't, but your body and mind crave it anyway. If you can resist it, this sensation fades and it even gets easier to resist. If you can't resist the pull, this particular anxiety, then only goes away when the relief of satisfying your craving is met. After someone gives in to the pull and stops denying getting to that satisfaction, the quicker the apprehension that shows up inside of you as anxiety of doing something you know you shouldn't do, not only goes away but eventually isn't even present, is when you have managed to develop a bigger problem. Instead, it is replaced with a different feeling of anxiety. Anxiety of not being able to get it again, or soon enough, after what will seem like a momentary high as you run out or just get low on your supply. This fear of being cut off, or even the fear of going through withdrawals, are two of the main reasons people who get hooked on hardcore drugs commit crimes to continue to get high. But it is a misconception. If you are going to get high, and you want to continue to get high, you need to go through the entire experience to its conclusion. Or rather you need to be able to.

Tom Petty sang that "coming down is the hardest part." He was singing about love, but if that song was secretly about drugs, coming down is not only the hardest part, it's the most necessary. As long as you can come down, on your own, and can abstain without fiending, you're all good. If you can't, discontinue, and seek professional help immediately. I'm not saying it's easy, I'm saying it is necessary, and taking sabbaticals can be pivotal.

What I'm talking about is a more disciplined approach to not only doing drugs, but taking medications, and anything else in life that can be abused, which let's face it, is just about everything. This also applies to sexaholics, alcoholics, work-aholics, exercise-aholics, electronic-aholics, etc.

Rule Five: The Law is the Law

If you partake in recreational substances again, keep in mind, the illegal ones are illegal for a reason, mostly. The legal ones are legal in certain areas for a reason again, mostly. Mainly, the powers that be in those areas stopped being ignorant about a prohibition that never should've been. At the same time, some areas have gone too far and found out the hard way that not all drugs, or all drug use, should be legal. And very little of any of it makes any sense whatsoever, let alone common sense. But one thing that is certain, it is exponentially harder to get high when you're locked up, and impossible if you're dead.

Also keep in mind, a lot of street drugs started as medication. Even meth. Methamphetamines, a.k.a. Crystal Meth, was invented by the Nazis as a performance enhancing drug called Pervitin. It is directly responsible for their massive early success at the beginning of World War II. And an integral part of using the war tactic called a Blitzkrieg. They could press on for days, and even weeks, overwhelming much of Europe, with the aid of Pervitin. It was also a major contributing factor to their blunders, and eventual loss of World War II after a certain point. And thank God, but why? Because meth is absolutely one of those few drugs that will completely ruin your life. It will warp your mind and make you paranoid beyond any resemblance of rationality. While at the same time giving you mass delusions of grandeur in all that you do, and it will not allow you to see that you actually fucked everything up.

One of the few times I did meth, actually the second time, I was seventeen. I ended up back at home later that evening (much later), to give the appearance of going to sleep and getting up in the morning. With the simple act of going into my room for more than a few hours and emerging in the morning during an hour that wouldn't raise any suspensions. I ended up just sketching all night. I drew a high contrast silhouette-esque portrait of Jim Morrision, the lead singer of The Doors, my favorite band from the 1960s. I'm not too shabby when it comes to art. A step or two above stick figures, anyway. As I copied his portrait onto paper in my own style, I found myself bursting with confidence and pride. This was certainly one of the best drawings I have ever done in my life. I was sure of it. The more progress I made that night, the better it looked. After a few hours I finally finished, and that was probably an hour, more or less, than I was actually aware of, as meth warps your sense of the passage of time as well. I tried to get a little sleep, which I did manage, but only barely. When I woke up, I excitedly grabbed my newest artistic creation to see it again, this time with the fresh eyes of first thing in the morning, which also meant sober.

I hadn't really done a Jim Morrison portrait as much as Mr. Ed. Yes, Mr. Ed, the talking TV horse originating from way back in the days of black and white television. I mean it was sort of Jim Morrison. If Jim had an eight-inch nose. But as I said, meth and few other hardcore drugs warp your perception (some medications included). In reality, too much of anything has that potential. And meth gives you itty bitty balls…just kidding, that's anabolic steroids. Most of the other hardcores will leave you needing oxygen, toothless (most of the time), impotent, and limp. But long-term side effects aside, not only did I have a misconception as to how well my drawing was turning out, but while I was in the midst of creating it, I had a massive sense of superiority and mastery, that after the fact, was also clearly a chemical delusion. And sure, it felt good to have that much confidence, but it wasn't real. Now, imagine those horrible side effects amplified and multiplied by months and even years of use. Ironically, as I write my book, the government downgraded marijuana from being classified as a Schedule 1 drug, which is as dangerous as heroin, PCP, and a few others, to being classified as a Schedule 3 drug which is only as bad as steroids. You're getting closer…or should I say warmer? Legalize marijuana medically and perhaps recreationally. If not, at least decriminalize recreational use. Put it into law that marijuana is not to ever be in large corporate hands, directly or indirectly. They will ruin it like they did tobacco and the medical field. Keep it in the hands of people who care. And make the hardcore drugs so illegal that no one will dare touch them.

One of the ways drugs warps someone's perception is convincing those of us that have done them, that they should all be legal. They shouldn't. The states of Washington and Oregon are learning this now. Another way drugs melt people's perception is when the drive to satisfy an addiction is so strong that the realities of doing hardcore street drugs are right out in the open, instead of behind closed doors. Currently, you see streets full of fentanyl junkies strung along this city street or that one, for blocks, now in every major and minor U.S. city. People who want that high so badly that they don't care how they get it, where they do it, how they live, or who sees it. People tranqed out, bodies flayed on sidewalks and street corners, crumpled in the corners of buildings and pavements, like casually discarded litter. Looking like the boneless chickens at The Far Side's Boneless Chicken Ranch. Only with human beings, piss, fecal matter, and dirty used syringes all over, instead of a funny joke with rubber chickens. The reality of this should at least put a crack in the delusion that all drugs should be legal, they shouldn't.

You need to understand that if you choose to do illegal street drugs, especially the hardcore ones, you are in the wrong. Not the law, not the cops. And most people do understand this, even if in a very primitive, subconscious way. Being an addict isn't a disease. It is more of a choice than anyone is willing to admit. Diseases you have to live with, addictions can be broken, beat, and overcome. Even though at times it may seem an insurmountable obstacle, it is not. This is where you stop making excuses.

So, in order to do drugs at all, break less laws by following all the other laws. Don't drink/drug and drive. And as previously mentioned, don't lie, cheat, or steal so you can do, or get drugs. And if you do drugs in public, keep it on the down low. There are a lot of folks who are perfectly happy not seeing or knowing about it. Most of those same people will drop a dime on you as soon as you show them otherwise. And, most importantly, don't do the wrong drugs. So that you can get high, continue to do so, and not die, or lose your piece of the pie.

Ask yourself, would people have a problem with drug use if no innocent bystanders were caught in the middle? If it were no different than drinking alcohol responsibly? And how much does someone care, who doesn't know, because they don't see?

Despite how the media sometimes paints law enforcement, they are not enemies. They are human beings, which means there are a few that are corrupt, but not all of them. Very few, in fact, cross that line. But like any group of human beings, there are always those who will abuse the system. Sadly, it's a part of the human condition. Most will uphold the law and do the right thing. Some will abuse their situation for their own selfish gains. So, here's the deal, this is the talk my father and mother gave to me as soon as I was old enough to hear it. They made sure I listened as soon as I was old enough to run into the police. That's run into, not run from. Don't run from the police, it will only make it worse. And "I was scared," never works as a defense for running and trying to evade the law. If you're wondering how old "old enough" is, if your kids are old enough to be out in public without you, aside from being dropped off, and picked up from school, that's how old.

My mother and father sat me down. My father, no stranger to being on the wrong side of the law, and my mother having heartbreakingly witnessed a fair share, if not most, of his trials going against the grain. Their dissertation went like this. "You need to respect the law and law enforcement. Police officers are only doing their jobs, and like it or not, it is an important job and one of the hardest jobs that is out there. If you get pulled over, or an officer stops you on the street, or anywhere, to speak with you for any reason, their first priority is their personal safety. They have their own life. Their own families, and their own friends. They want and expect to go home every day, same as everyone else with any other job. They want to see their loved ones at the end of each, and every day, same as everyone else. So, first and foremost, be compliant. When they tell you to do something, you do it, no questions or excuses. If you say anything you best watch your tone, be respectful by using common courtesy, and use "sir" or "ma'am" if it's a female officer. Do not be a smartass, and do not speak unless spoken to. Be straightforward and direct when you answer their questions. Use as few words as you have to, and without volunteering information. Under no circumstances do you try to assault, resist, hit, fight, or run from the police. They have the legal right to shoot you in most of those situations, and if you cross that line, they will be in the right to do so. And as your parents, there is nothing we can do about it because you were in the wrong."

It can feel heavy when your own parents tell you the reality equivalent of "fuck around and find out the hard way," is simply how it is. But it was the brutally honest talk all parents should have with their children. Notice how my parents told me that the police will shoot me to protect themselves and protect others, but they didn't say it's because of your skin color? Just checking, and I'm not saying that it doesn't happen some of the time, I'm saying that most of the time it is justified and 100% preventable with a little compliance. So, if you or someone you know and love earned it, you damn well also know it, own it.

As I mentioned earlier, you don't sacrifice your friendships, or other relationships, to get drugs or to do them. You don't lie, cheat, or steal to get drugs. If you justify any of that to get high, you have a problem. You do not commit any act of violence to get drugs, or for drugs in any way, shape, or form. Doing drugs recreationally should be as much about coming together and finding common ground as any other positive social situation. They aren't seen that way because of the few that involve violence and/or take it to a level of violence when drugs are concerned and involved. Alcohol can have that effect as well, but it isn't viewed the same because alcohol has been legal for long enough that it has been seen and proven that it can be imbibed without everything else getting out of control.

Lucky Luciano, Al Capone's mentor, had it right in the middle of prohibition. There is no need for the violence, as violence is bad for "business." And there is more than enough "business" to go around. Where they, and their Irish criminal counterparts, screwed the pooch (or in this case hooch), was getting violent in the first place, and continuing to do so. But the

St. Valentine's Day Massacre, on the order of Al Capone, in retaliation for the Irish mob's betrayal of his boss, was when the authorities took notice, and they knew someone had to take action. Because of the sheer level of shock and awe violence. It was too much for normal folks to stomach even though it was out of retaliation. Would Chicago, although still notorious for crime and corruption, be worse, better, or just a different criminal haven today had that not happened? Perhaps if they could've gotten the Irish Mob to work with them, Chicago would possibly only be known for lesser crimes and corruption, instead of one of the murder and criminal capitals of the world. Say what you want about the Mafia and other well put together criminal organizations, the ones worth their salt, typically keep the violence in certain neighborhoods to a minimum and amongst themselves, away from innocents, because they know it draws unwanted attention. Attention that is bad for business. When things get violent, extortion insurance scams included, that's when the authorities start to notice and it all begins to unravel. If innocent people aren't involved, the law doesn't get involved. As far as attracting unwanted attention is concerned, it's bad for business in legal commerce as well. When people get taken advantage of in the wrong way, and for long enough, again, it catches the eye of unwanted attention and leads to more government regulations. If you want less government oversight, quit screwing over your customers, clients, and patients. If everyone gets a fair deal, there is no reason for anyone to feel cheated, there is no reason for harsh feelings, and there is no reason to involve regulatory agents, people, or organizations.

In the movie "American Gangster" we know that everyone loved Frank Lucas. Those who lived around him anyway. The notorious Frank Lucas was "Bumpy" Johnson's righthand man before he took over. He was loved by people who knew him and lived in his neighborhood because he took care of the people in his neighborhood and organization. We know Capone was also loved in a similar way for similar reasons. The public outcry comes after something heinous starts. And it never comes from those who are also benefiting. It comes from those who have lost and suffered, and sometimes it comes from someone who witnesses it going too far. No one would even know who or what cartels or even the mafia are, if violence had never been involved in the first place. And let's be honest, if there is no violence or additional crime involved, even a drug addict becomes less of a daunting thing, and more on the level of a nonviolent alcoholic. And that brings us to our next rule…

Rule Six: The Line in the Sand

Look, a certain number of people are going to do drugs, just like a certain number of people are going to drink. Not everyone who takes drugs has a problem with being addicted to drugs. Just like not everyone who drinks is an alcoholic. When people take issue with other people doing drugs or drinking alcohol is when the line that is darkness, gets crossed out in the open, right in front of everyone. It is when lines of human decency are desecrated. It is when innocent people get caught in a crossfire. It is when too many people get hurt or too many people die, and let's be honest, one overdose is too many. All make for big problems that are harder and harder to deny. Again, would you have a problem with someone else's drug use if it was no different than enjoying an alcoholic beverage responsibly? And what happens if the cartels, drug dealers, middlemen, and users all stop with the violence and start cooperating? Does anyone really have a problem with someone doing drugs if no one was ever killed, hurt, or stolen from?

Look, I get it. All that glitters is gold. The good life really does look good, and it can be if it's done the right way. If it isn't, the things you own will not only end up owning you, but when you do lose them, or they get taken away, it is devastating because you thought you had it, you feel like you came so far, and thus you fell even further. But the reality is you took shortcuts, and you had the delusion of ownership when you were really on a ticking countdown to lose it all. That is when you find out that you were only renting, so you didn't really achieve any kind of tangible wealth, as true wealth that is earned honestly cannot be taken away so easily.

A note to the cartels, mafia, gangs, and every other form of organized crime, as well as modern day businesses and corporations who have decided to emulate these poor examples. A culture of greed, violence, death, and financial inequality is only tolerated for a time. There will come a point of reckoning for anyone perpetrating these monstrosities. History has shown us this time and time again. Those who hurt and oppress and take advantage of others eventually will come to know justice. Those who perpetrated a culture of corruption will eventually reap what you sow. Whether that is a cohort's betrayal, an opposition's assassination, a shift in business trends that your company can't keep up with, or the long arm of the law, it will eventually happen. What I am talking about is business 101, adapt or perish. If you continue to take advantage of, hurt, and kill your customers. And you continue to hurt and kill your competition, and they continue to do the same, and you hurt and kill each other within your own organization as well as your customers, it will come to an end or be put to an end. Everything must evolve, and that includes evolving beyond degradation. It is time.

Furthermore, doing drugs, or rather being under the influence of drugs, cannot be an excuse for aberrant behavior any longer. It should be considered indefensible to rationalize indiscretion because of momentary intoxication. It is one of those not-so-clever lies that law enforcement eventually catches on to. It is only a matter of time before the prosecution, courts, and the general public, does as well.

Again, let's dispel the rumors. Cops are human beings. There are good ones and there are a few that are just plain bad. Same as almost anywhere, almost any group, and almost any occupation. I'd love to tell you that someone who gets into law enforcement only does so for the right reasons, and none of them ever become corrupted, but that's not reality. Reality is a human being is a human being. For the most part, cops are not only trying to do the very difficult yet noble job of "protect and serve," but also a necessary and often thankless one. It was Thomas Paine who wrote Common Sense. It is basically a dissertation as to why government and laws are necessary evils as mankind can be selfishly destructive towards each other. It also warns of the dangers of too much government, as well as too much government overreach, during a time when this nation, America, was being shaped. He notes, and much more eloquently than this, that, if mankind could be trusted to be conscionable, government wouldn't be necessary. But, because mankind cannot be trusted to do the right thing, an overseer entity, like a government, becomes a necessary evil. For what I'm trying to convey the end result translates to, hence you bring it on yourself and others when you cross a certain line, but especially when you cross it repeatedly.

Understand there is no such thing as street cred. If there was, no one who wanted to be a career criminal would try to avoid jail. All higher-ups in criminal organizations would even do their own time instead of handing it down, like a coward, to their subordinates, and no one would even run from the cops. If street cred was a real thing, you would blatantly go and commit a crime and turn yourself in, if you couldn't get arrested on the spot. It is the stupidest thing to think that doing time makes you a real or even a better criminal. In reality, it makes you a fucking billboard, a beacon to point out the rest of the law breakers to law enforcement. It's called guilty by association, and it makes doing illegal business under the radar much harder, if not almost impossible, at times. Which should be the goal. See no evil, hear no evil, speak no evil.

I really feel like this saying can be taken a couple of ways. For those of you who don't realize it, this saying can be more about staying away from bad things, so they don't corrupt you. If you aren't exposed to seeing or hearing bad things, you are less likely to do or say bad things yourself. Which isn't a bad philosophy.

Hear no evil, see no evil, speak no evil. First, my more nefarious interpretation. If you're going to do something wrong and you want to get away with it, you let no one see you, and you don't tell anyone, thus no one hears about it. If nobody knows, it becomes a kind of "it's only wrong if you get caught" philosophy. Or, if no one knows a crime was committed, did it occur? Similar to a tree falling in the forest when no one is around to hear it.

And a more practical but equally shady version. If you have to keep a secret, tell no one. Unless you have to tell someone else, in which case you might be screwed anyway. But in this instance, we will take "hear no evil, see no evil, speak no evil" to mean if people don't see it or hear about it, they can't drop a dime about it. And literally don't care about it. Because how can you care about what you don't know? If you're a cartel leader or member, and your organization is so violent that your fellow country men and women and children are leaving your country in droves, it means your entire group failed to stay under the radar and thus have exposed yourself and your entire operation. Turning it into a carton of milk with a currently expired expiration date, rather than a time enduring organization carved from marble.

As I have mentioned, my father was a bit of a bastard. Of course, he wasn't the absolute worst that humanity has to offer, but there have been many more who were better men than him, than those who were worse. Despite that he, on occasion, gave very good advice. Reinforcing my theory that sometimes wisdom can come from some not-so-wise places. "Hands at ten and two, thumbs up, check mirrors and gauges every two-three seconds. A defensive driver always knows their surroundings." He'd bark at me like a drill sergeant, whether we were in a vehicle or not. And "No son, you don't want to be anything like me, be better." Which was probably the single best advice he gave me. But the most relevant advice he gave me for the purpose of this book is, "Don't do the crime, if you can't do the time." Time served is hard time, and full of violence. To top that off, the sex you want, you won't get, the sex you don't want, you will get. And that's sugar coating it.

Aside from the violence that nobody should want (in or out of prison), from a money-making perspective, violence is bad for business and doesn't help propagate repeat customers or true loyalty from your cohorts. If you know the people you work for, or are doing business with, will kill you if things go sideways, it commands no loyalty. Fear is not loyalty or respect; It is a metaphorical ticking time bomb.

Don't advertise. If you have a shirt that says "stoner," and a tattoo of a pot leaf on your forearm, yeah, the cops are going to get to know you as soon as they see you. Just like the song, only in a way that you won't like or want. So, let's call it the wrong way. It's cool to have a personal style, but if you look like a duck, walk like a duck, and talk like a duck, don't be surprised if you get shot during hunting season. This is where you need to tone it down a bit because it's always open season on drug users year-round, for many reasons. And keep in mind the only people who don't work the graveyard shift but are up and about, through the wee hours of the evening and morning, are typically up to no good. It is another red flag, and law enforcement will know something is up. Expect this and take the correct precautions and preparations between the hours of 11:00 pm and 5:00 am. As in, don't be seen through those hours. Be somewhere you can stay during that time frame. Or at least, don't be riding dirty. If you're not breaking the law, you can't get caught breaking the law.

Rule Seven: Keep it Local and Ethical

Only deal with people you trust, people who don't do stupid things, people who themselves have standards. Loyalty, and yes, morals. If you get caught, take responsibility for it, and never let someone else take the fall for something you did. That is pure cowardice. It's called, "owning it." If you do end up having to do time, keep in mind that you are the one who screwed up. The consequences are usually less when you own it, instead of denying it. While you are serving your time, paying your dues, it's okay to communicate with the outside world, and even ask for a little help, but when you ask too much, you are interrupting someone else's life on the outside, when you're the one who is inside, locked up, not okay. You don't try to make other people do your time with you. It is a matter of not taking advantage of others, and realizing that life did not stop for them when you went in. On the contrary, life kept going, 100% unabated by your fuck up. By default, life goes on, no matter what, leaving some people behind.

But how do we know who to trust? Who deserves loyalty? I would recommend the merit system, the way the samurai described it. How to know loyalty in a person, or rather, why to know loyalty in a person. In Bushido Sho

Shinshu, The Way of The Samurai, it describes one of its principles referred to as "Remembering Your Debts." It isn't that you owe the mortgage company or your landlord "X" amount of dollars each month. It isn't that your tab is due at your local bar, and you did or didn't pay it. It isn't even the ten grand you owe your bookie (and hopefully you don't). It is remembering what others do for you and have done for you. That way you know who you can count on, both in good times and in bad ones. It is also a way to surround yourself with quality people, thus helping yourself to become a more quality individual as well. It will show you who you can lean on in tough times, and who should be able to lean on you in their respective hardships (and they will all be deeply personal, no matter how similar). Make no mistake, this is also how you show others your value, your quality as a human being. From the same perspective, it can also show you who not to associate with as well. In an ideal world everyone could lean on everyone. Alas, people are just as corruptible as paper is susceptible to water. The trick is don't get wet (but maybe that only works if you are paper).

Know that a stranger is a stranger until they have earned it, thoroughly earned it, and not with violence. It's a lot harder to prove loyalty without forcing someone to commit a crime or even kill for you. That's the easy way to instill fear and gain leverage over someone, not earn loyalty. Earning loyalty without required violence might be the more difficult path, but it is also the path that leads to stronger, more productive bonds that are truly fruitful. Know that real loyalty isn't forced, or coerced, and thus cannot be lost as easily. If it is forced, or coerced, it can simply be lost at any given time.

If your so-called "friend" is dealing drugs and slips a hot load in his stash to up his sales, he's a murderer, and thus, not trustworthy. And anyone who would seek out drugs that someone else OD'd on, is stupid and suicidal. That doesn't mean that it is the good stuff, it means that it is the bad stuff from the wrong kind of people. If you die, you can't continue to get high, dummy!

Part of the problem, for the longest time is, if someone does illegal street drugs a certain amount, personal depravity is assumed and even expected from an outsider's perspective. Similar to telling someone they are one day way more likely to try, and become addicted, to high level street narcotics because they smoked marijuana. Now, does someone really have an inevitability of trying harder drugs simply because they smoked marijuana? Or does the suggestion of one heading down a path that leads to another, and another, and another, until an unavoidable doom of unrestricted drug use and depravity hold influence over someone's psyche? Or is this again, a choice? I've known plenty of people that only smoked pot. Or people who only did drugs that are classified as natural by the drug user community. Like marijuana, alcohol, and mushrooms. Very few of them took it too far. At the same time, I have known those who constantly sought the next high, a better high, a more prolific high. Or even sought that constant drunk. Some of them are alive today, but I can't tell you they went down that path simply because they decided to try marijuana one day. I happen to know one individual whose first drug was L.S.D., not even alcohol. I can't imagine how intense that was. I will tell you that if you can use drugs without getting out of control might very well be dependent on what drugs you use or even the amount, but at the same time, I've never been so high on anything that I didn't know right from wrong, so maybe the depravity associated with dope is also much more of a choice than everyone tends to believe.

So, we set some manners for drug use. As an example we'll use pot, grass, doja, marijuana, mary jane, or my favorite (because it is so grossly inaccurate and over one-hundred years old at this point) the devil's weed. But, keep in mind, most of these rules are interchangeable with other drugs as well as many activities. First, never force or trick someone into doing drugs, not even marijuana, or anything else for that matter. Drug use should only be voluntary and by free will, and hopefully with a little honest education. When smoking in a group, contribute if you can. It's called "matching" or "pitching in" when you're smoking pot. But really, no matter what you're doing, it's only polite to at least bring some green bean casserole to the potluck. If you can't throw in this time, don't expect anyone to match you next time. Although, if you're cool, you will not always care about someone matching you. Because, if you're cool, you understand that not everybody is always able to pitch in, and drugs have no real value. However, know that if you are the person that never kicks in, people take notice. And that's one of the reasons you should know that recreational drugs, like alcohol even, are mostly meant to be social and in a positive way. When you start to treat drugs with an avarice attitude, you're developing a problem. Then whatever you're doing, whether it is drinking, speeding, banging, burning, or anything else, it has become a problem. At that point, it has been controlling you and warping your behavior and consciousness, and it will continue to do so as long as your number one priority is to achieve your specific and preferred endorphin release.

Let's keep it down to earth and realistic about consuming weed. It is a drug. Drugs should not have any actual value attached to them, so let's be more practical in how we smoke it in a waste not, want not, sort of way. If you don't waste it, then you're not also wasting other resources to get more, like time, money, and even fuel. My first pot smoking experience was Martin Luther King Jr. Day, 1995. My best friend and I smoked some Mexican brick weed out of a brass fitting with a screen. The screen was also brass. Procured from his mother's bathroom faucet and placed precariously in the bottom of the wide part of the brass nipple fitting. That served as our makeshift amateur bowl. It was crude, but it worked. As the years passed, we continued our juvenile delinquency behavior and swiftly became more regular consumers and, as such, we advanced to being more sophisticated smokers. We both eventually paid up for our own chamber pipes. A chamber pipe was made of brass, but with a nickel-plated silver finish on the outside with some parts having a metallic oil on water sheen to them. The entire chamber pipe unscrewed section by section to make cleaning it and scraping it on those dry days easier, along with one larger chamber, usually located in the middle of the stem, where some of us would put a single bud. We would keep that lone bud in the chamber and let it get resinated, as we smoked our pot through the chamber pipe. Eventually removing the resinated nugget and smoking it for an "added" effect.

The more people I met and smoked with, the more I came to realize that a lot of people had their own personal smoking preferences. So much so that some people even differentiated themselves with their smoking apparatus, as some people do with cars or clothing. Some used corn cob pipes, like General Douglas McArthur. While others preferred a cheap plastic Graffix Bong (they were hard to carry with you, and even harder to conceal. A big concern when it was still 100% illegal). Some used their father's old opium pipe that was brought back from Vietnam. There were pipes carved from rock, antler, or wood for the naturalist enthusiast, or even a peace pipe. Not an antique peace pipe, but a newly made one, and yes, they do still make them. That was all a small farm town in a still hidden and isolated corner of Colorado had in the mid-1990s, until my friends and I discovered the wonderful world of glass pipes.

That was around the same time we, as a society, seemed to enter what I refer to as an age of extreme decadence. Cell phones that are as small as watches, ironically, eventually becoming watches. To cell phones the size of an open Stephen King novel, not as thick, yet has access to exponentially more information and stories than fit in one of Mr. King's novels. Ipods, jewelry that isn't limited to being adornments anymore, now it's electronic health tracking bling. You can also accessorize yourself from the inside out with Botox, Restylane, tattooed permanent makeup, breast and butt implants. Or indulge in half-million-dollar vehicles, when there are businessmen and women so rich, they're now famous for it. While tv and movie stars are idolized instead of first responders, who are socially crucified in the name of profit, politics, and propaganda. But for the purpose of this discussion, let's keep it simple for now and back on a more relevant topic, pipes.

I'm certainly guilty of indulging in the age of decadence, as most of us are to some degree. And how can you not be? Unless you are a monk in a monastery, it's hard not to get swept up in this fast-paced-give-me-everything-instantly-society. It is constantly thrown in our face. I was especially guilty when it came to pipes, as were more than a few of us. It was 1996, I was sixteen when I graduated from my brass chamber pipe to my first color changing glass pipe. I can still describe it perfectly. It was, of course, all glass with a perfectly straight neck in between the bowl and the mouthpiece. Three raised strips of glass began on the tube neck, near the top of the bowl, and curved clockwise around the neck down to the mouthpiece, ending in a similar manner as a barber's pole is striped. The mouthpiece was a slightly larger diameter than the neck/stem to form a definitive mouthpiece. The glass bubble, that hosted the bowl, was also perfectly round, except for a slight flat spot on the bottom, so it could sit on a flat surface and not roll away, and of course the indentation that formed the bowl. The pipe was colored with an iridescent yellow when it was clean, and a magnificent blue and white that rivaled a bright blue sky, streaked with white clouds, spread thin across the skyscape when the inside was coated with a black background that was the leftover resin from incinerated marijuana smoke rushing through the pipe, eventually accumulating a black coating on every surface the smoke grazes across. The carb, or carburetor, was on the left side of the bowl as you looked down the pipe from the mouthpiece. The whole thing was about four inches long. It was my first and, respectively, my favorite.

It was one of those favorites, not necessarily because it was my first, but a favorite because of the memories attached to it. My childhood best friend, Sonny, went over one-thousand miles away for the summer of 1997, ironically to a place called Runaway Bay, TX (or as stoners like to call Texas, Hell. And you'll find out why in a minute) with his father, Mr. Vale. He was the auto mechanics teacher at our local high school. One of Mr. Vale's favorite students, a young man by the name of Tad, also went with them. Tad was two years older than Sonny and I, who were only a month and a half apart, and Tad was already with offspring. I hadn't met Tad yet, but we would eventually come to be close friends as well.

One day Sonny calls me, his voice seeped in desperation, "Dude, you gotta help me! I can't find weed anywhere! We can find meth everywhere, and every color of the rainbow too! But no one has any weed!" (Which is why we called it Hell, no other reason than a whole lot of the wrong drugs and not enough of the right ones.) He briefly pauses, almost as if to catch his breath. "If you send me some weed, I'll hook you up with a glass pipe when we come back." He had to do some talking, and more bargaining, but I eventually, yet hesitantly, agreed.

So I procured a half-ounce, triple bagged it with brand name double sealing freezer bags, and placed it in the middle of a "handmade candle" that I made from melting a bunch of leftover candle corpses (those are the remaining bits of wax from candles after a wick has burned all the way down and failed to melt the last of the wax) together in one of my mom's old pots on her kitchen stove and poured it into a wide mouth quart mason jar, the half-ounce, of course, encased in the middle. When you're out of pot and you want some, the feeling is called Jonesing. It's different from a junkie fiend, it can be resisted, and it doesn't have an urgent panic of getting the craving satisfied.

Until you let it. If you do need to discontinue marijuana, you will only get a little grumpy for a maximum of thirty to forty-five days, if you don't also do a body flush regiment. And that's exactly who I sent it to. Ben Joansen, in Texas, through an anonymous package service. Not realizing my friend was lusting for it, putting too much priority on it, as well as its value. He said when he got it, he had to chase the package courier down. The courier didn't think it was a legitimate person, and he was right. After retrieving the package and the courier drove away, Sonny promptly ripped open the box and slammed the mason jar on the concrete, shattering it and the candle that I had poured my heart and soul into making (not really, more like thirty minutes) and immediately pulled out the weed.

Not too long after getting my first pipe was when I became another proud proprietor of a plethora of paraphernalia. I had bongs, chillums, traditional pipes, sherlocks, bubblers, shotguns, and the list goes on. Each with their own qualities and purposes. Some smooth, others harsh, some even harsh on purpose. After all, if you smoke out of something that is called a "shotgun," don't expect for it to feel nice…until it does. Some pieces were for show with color changing glass, others made a bit more practical, concealable, and durable. Some unconcealable and big, but water cooled, others so bold and harsh you only need one hit, of course that one hit was the equivalent of more than a few joints, give or take.

But back to the manners of consuming marijuana. When smoking in a group, pass it to the left biddy-bum-bum. This way no one feels favored. And don't be the person who always sits, or tries to sit, on the left of whomever is about to light the joint. FYI, it's usually the person rolling it, providing the weed for it, or has the fire for it. Pot provider's pick. Similar to a dealer's pick in poker. In my group, if you tried to sit on the left of whomever you thought was going to light and hit it first, we would intentionally switch up who got "greens" with, "Alright, it's rolled now (or packed in the event of a bowl). Who's got some fire?" (slang for a lighter) That way it started in a totally different unexpected place. Sit where you can, and if available sit where you can be comfortable. On a recreational level, weed especially, should be a social event.

And from that same aspect, don't take a scavenger hit. If you're smoking a bowl versus a joint or blunt, spark the flame on your lighter next to the bowl, slowly bring the flame closer to the edge of the bowl as you gently inhale until the flame curves over the edge, barely touching the smallest fraction of the greens, singeing only a small portion on the top of the bowl. Quickly remove the fire as soon as a cherry is established, but before too much of the weed is burnt.

Unless you're using a chillum or a variation of a chillum, a quality glass pipe will have a carburetor. This is because marijuana smoke goes stale very quickly. After you have either filled the apparatus like a bong, or a reasonably sized glass pipe, with smoke, rather you fill it all the way or partially, release your finger from the carb on a pipe, or bong, or pull the bowl out for a slide carb (in the case of a slide carb. Water pipe) and inhale the smoke, making sure to inhale the rest (or most) of the smoke, clearing the pipe or smoking apparatus. Stale marijuana smoke will make you cough, and not in a good way, especially stale smoke in a bong. Hence it is good manners to clear the pipe, or other smoking apparatus, before passing it on, and good manners by not wasting. After you inhale, check to make sure the pipe is clear, if it isn't already from releasing that carb. Do this by either blowing some fresh air through it with the carb unencumbered or clearing it by inhaling the remainder of the idle smoke. If you get a pipe that still has stale smoke in, give a puff of fresh air through it to clear it yourself, but don't make a big deal about it. Not all smoking apparatuses are created equal, and most have a particular drawback or two.

From here, as a group or individually, you have two choices. Either keep the cherry going without using any additional flame, just good old oxygen fed embers, or lightly tamp it out with slight but constant pressure using the bottom edge of a lighter, a tamping device, or man up and use the tip of your finger or thumb. It'll only hurt until it doesn't, or until the cherry is out. Snuffing it out by depriving it of oxygen can also be a viable method. The next person (to the left!) does the same thing, if there is no cherry ember and it needs to be relit, once again, take as little of the greens as possible while using as little flame from the lighter as possible. Allowing you to still get a taste of the fresh greens and trying to leave a taste for the next person and not igniting too much of the marijuana. The next person either tries to keep a cherry going or relights it, then lightly tamps it out. Hopefully, everyone you smoke with gets a taste of the greens. If a second or even third bowl is loaded for the same group in the same smoking session, whoever got the cashed hit from the last bowl, gets first "greens" on the next bowl. Again, so nobody feels like they always get the hit that tastes like ass. Not literally, it is called the ass hit because it is the tail end of the bowl and has a definitive bad taste compared to the rest of the bowl, and the ash in the bottom of the bowl can also pull all of the way through the pipe, giving an additional ass taste, unless you need to clean your pipe and it was a deluge of dirty resin that was deposited in your mouth, extra ass taste. Unfortunately, it will inevitably and eventually happen unless you are consistent with cleaning your preferred smoking device. But seriously, using this slow smoking method, smoking for flavor, as opposed to everyone taking the biggest most prolific hit they can, a.k.a. being selfish scavengers, and you will notice that not only does everyone who is smoking the bowl gets higher with less, but it's also more enjoyable for the group and hence more enjoyable for each person involved.

Back in the 1990s we'd smoke the whole bowl that way for that reason. It goes a lot further, and everyone gets a lot higher. Another is etiquette, if not only everyone gets to taste a part of the good greens, and everyone takes turns in finishing the bowl down to the "waste-not-want-not" nitty gritty, no one feels left out or shorted. No one feels they intentionally and constantly get the shaft while someone else almost always benefits. Putting everyone on that same level, that same high (individual tolerances allowing for such). Being on the same level also makes for a better shared experience. No one likes a scavenger. One of the old school aspects is the "waste not want not" part. Marijuana wasn't always in such heavy supply as it is now. Legality will apparently increase availability. But I believe this one should be practiced first and foremost to keep from becoming too avarice or decadent with it. Back then it was either feast or famine, but you could always count on two "dry" times each year, spring and late fall/early winter, which was right before and after snowboarding season. I honestly never thought I would see the day when marijuana became legal, but I still think we're one stupid asshole away from having it ruined for the rest of us. In the states where marijuana is legal, it is similar to a fragile peace treaty that not everyone is onboard with.

Again, keep in mind that recreationally, a positive social atmosphere where people are doing drugs together, always helps the experience, especially when everyone is on the same level, and with the same high. Don't camp on the bowl, pipe, or joint, and know it is not a microphone. Honestly, this one is more of a lightweight, "forgot I was holding it because I'm stoned, faux pas." Once you get high, put it aside, and do something. If you're only smoking pot, and it ends with simply being so high that you can't even change the channel, or get off of the couch, so you watch a horrible show and eat an entire bag of chips, what was the difference from doing heroin, and laying in a dark alley, or on a grungy street, through your entire high? One example of why you need to do something and why you shouldn't just sit there high. There is a huge difference, but not from an outsider's perspective. Doing drugs, the right drugs, should be an experience enhancer. Not an experience on its own. Play ping-pong, a board game, or Twister. Have a conversation, watch a movie, or conquer a video game. Smoke a "J" right before going on a walk or even a hike. But do something, and with your friends.

Don't get me wrong, get your legs under you first. Absolutely everyone turns into such a giggly little girl that they're worthless the first few times that they drink (but in a silly fun way). Drugs are no different in that aspect. It takes a minute to learn how to handle your booze, or weed, or dope, or medication for that matter. Be honest, up until reading my book, have you ever honestly considered alcohol a drug? It is. What about tobacco? Also is. Caffeine? That Starbucks Grande morning rocket boost shouldn't seem so innocent now. Most people don't realize this, or don't want to, but all should. How about that prescription your doctor writes to help alter your mood or aid in sleep? We need to be more aware of what we put in our bodies by realizing the similarities between hardcore street drugs and prescription medications only begins with each being chemical compounds but also the similarities are nearly endless, good and bad. However or whatever you choose to do, make a ritual out of it and a positive one. Especially if you use it medically.

Rule Eight: Knowledge is Power

The most dangerous thing about drugs is the misinformation that exists, and has existed, about many of them for longer than prohibition has been imposed on any of them. I have met many people in my life. People who are very poor and people who are very wealthy. People who lived with inward posterity and people who basked in material riches. And yes, there is a difference.

The ones I've known who eventually, or immediately, became hooked on hardcore street drugs at some time all expressed the same, or similar, thought, no matter what their lifestyle or stature. "If they lied to me about something as harmless as pot (marijuana), what else did they lie to me about?" The more you know the safer you'll be, not to say drugs are safe by any means. They aren't (even the medical ones, shh!). And how do you know what good advice is and what bad advice is, when it comes to something that was lied about in the first place from sources that you are supposed to be able to trust? If something, or someone, like an organization or authority figure lied a lot, or even a little bit to begin with, it makes it difficult to trust any information about any of it, especially from that same, now discredited source. That's one of many reasons why I decided to write this book. Unlike some cartoon heroes from the eighties, I do not have the power of the universe. I do however have some pivotal and crucial answers, and it would be immoral to not share what I have learned, know, and practice on a daily basis. The fact of the matter is drugs are dangerous, and drugs can kill. Even when you know what you're doing, and even when you get them from someone who is supposed to be trustworthy and knows what they are doing. But, a little bit of wisdom goes a long way, and has the potential to keep us from making some serious mistakes most of the time. A little bit of the right knowledge keeps us from getting ripped off, keeps us away from the wrong drugs, keeps us aware of the possibility of addiction. It can keep us from buying low grade drugs and keeps us from dying or going to prison until it's all legal and even after that. And make no mistake, one day this whole drug business will be legal. As soon as the powers that be figure out how much money can be made from it all. The whole drug business. Not millions. Billions, even trillions and more. The trick is legalizing the right ones and getting rid of the wrong ones. While at the same time, learning to enjoy and appreciate what is reasonable with drug use, to avoid becoming unreasonable ourselves. And figuring out what is truly more beneficial than harmful with prescription medications.

So, how do you keep yourself and your friends safe? How do you keep from becoming unreasonable? The kind of unreasonableness that makes people justify crossing lines of ethics and acceptable human behavior. Lines like lying, cheating, stealing, killing, or even worse? And all in the name of getting that next high. Or using drugs as an excuse for committing abhorrent behavior, not even anything sustainable. Have proper perspective and don't do the wrong drugs.

Once again, here is one of the great paradoxes of people who have a hardcore addiction. People who not only cannot but admittedly refuse to even try to keep it under control, they become so intoxicated that they "fall off," and typically won't remember most of it, if any of it, making the entire event a waste. They get way too high, or way too drunk, to the point where they blackout. From the similar aspect of, "If a tree falls in the woods and no one is around to hear it, does it make a sound?" Only in this scenario it's, "If someone gets so high they don't even remember the experience, did they actually get high? Or was the attempt to get high a complete waste?" Only this one has a definitive answer, "hell yes it was a waste." Whatever they did, experienced, or whatever was done to them, isn't even real in their minds (if they remember it), and a lot of times it can be completely out of character for a sober version of themselves, so it makes those things that happened harder to accept happened, and thus impossible to process. While it still seems to leave an indelible ink stain on your subconscious and thus affects your entire psyche and life. Again, you don't let a substance control you. Or anything for that matter. But at the point that you consumed something that you have zero recollection, yet you have all of the physical and mental damage doing something like that causes, especially repeatedly, and with no memories, trophies, rewards, or payout. Because even if you had a trophy of an epic night that you don't remember, it would mean nothing without the memory and story that went with it. Thus, you not only wasted money and drugs, but your time and health as well.

In the mid-1980s, when I was a little kid, my best friend and I would try to whittle our days away, playing Nintendo video games. The gaming system that did what Atari couldn't do by taking video games from gimmicks and dark arcades in shopping malls, to mainstream entertainment in every home that could afford one, and many that couldn't. My mother would often make us shut it off and go outside to play. Every time she did, it came with the same lecture. I've included the original version and followed it up with a modified version, so it doesn't only apply to video games or movies/ television, but what I've been writing about all this whole time and a little more. I call it, The Nintendo Lecture.

The original lecture:

"You will not spend all of your time playing video games. It is a beautiful day. You and your friends need to go outside and play. Enjoy the day. Life is not in here or in that game box, life is out there. It isn't healthy to stare at that screen all day like zombies. You will not play that thing for hours at a time, let alone all day. It will melt your brain." Something most of our parents and grandparents and guardians, pretty much anyone who was older, would warn us about being a couch potato and watching too much tv or playing too many video games. "You can use it with moderation, but if I catch you sneaking in to play it, I will take it away. You also need to understand that real people, in real life, don't behave like that. If I catch your behavior changing in a bad or unconstructive way, I will take it away."

The modified lecture to fit any situation that lacks moderation:

"You should not spend all of your time doing that. It is beautiful outside, you as well as your friends need to go outside and enjoy the day. Life is not in here or in that, life is out there. It isn't healthy to do anything too much and it will turn you into zombies. You cannot do that for hours at a time let alone all day. Too much of anything is a bad thing and will adversely affect your brain and body to varying degrees. You can use it, or anything else, with moderation and never have a problem. But if you catch yourself being sneaky to do it, know that no one will take it away from you, you'll need to self-regulate. You also need to understand that real people, in real life, don't behave poorly. If your behavior changes in a bad or unconstructive way, you might want and need to reevaluate your habits."

It seemed ridiculous to hear The Nintendo Lecture out loud when back then, for so many people, how people behaved on television, movies, and especially video games, wasn't normal or acceptable behavior, was simply tacit and "For Entertainment Purposes Only." Now what parents and grandparents warned us about television and video games melting our brains and not only controlling us but raising our children and turning everyone into brain-dead zombies in the eighties, is all coming to complete fruition. Seriously, the next time you are in a group of people, look up from your phone or tablet, and observe everyone else in the room. Most likely all of them are intently staring at their phones/devices, aren't they? If you think this is what a group of friends doing drugs looks like, all focused, like brainwashed zombies on that one thing, you're half right. The big difference is that druggies talk to each other. And ironically, there is study, after study, about how excessive device time, including and especially social media, is counter-productive for a young maturing mind. But how many people have looked at how devastating it is for a docile mind, or even an aging one? I've witnessed it warp my friends, as well as my aging mother, after I experienced it manipulating me. I quit social media and had all of my accounts erased a long time ago and began to limit my personal device time when I noticed that "influence" in my life and my disposition has been better for it ever since. If you are reading my book on a digital platform, again, I do apologize for using the latest and greatest drug to bring it to you. It was simply my best outlet to reach the greatest number of people. If you like my book, and it helped you, or it offered a new perspective, and you wish to share it with other people, I would, once more, encourage you to please try to do so by buying a paper copy for a gift, or even for your own bookshelf. And if you can't, sharing it digitally is better than not sharing it at all.

Rule Nine: Don't Get Caught

My best friend and I received some quality advice when we were seventeen and both stood before a court of law for the first time. Wait, let me back-up. After a fun night of tripping acid (yes, I said tripping acid. As in L.S.D. Lysergic Acid Diethylamide), my best friend and I decided we would go buy some donuts for not only ourselves, but my mother as well, whose house we were staying at that night, and also snuck out from that previous evening to go have a good time as young people probably shouldn't, but sometimes do. After all, I held down two jobs and paid more than a few of my own bills and still managed to attend high school. No reason I can't buy a sugary breakfast for the household. Living in a small town that was beginning to bud in the mid-1990s, we decided to go to the new grocery store that had been open for business for less than a month. Being on "the flipside" of an acid trip, and in a brand new, very large store in our nothing-ever-happens-town, we decide to take the long way around the isles to the bakery, to take the full tour.

In hindsight, I should have thought it suspicious, every time we rounded a corner, I saw the same overzealous security guard behind us at the beginning of whatever aisle we were at the end of. Lurking just around the previous corner we had rounded. We had nothing nefarious in mind, other than an unhealthy breakfast for everyone, so I thought very little of the creepy man slinking around, that far behind us, like I said, until thinking back in hindsight, after all was said and done. When we rounded that last back corner of the store and had the bakery and donut shelves in sight, we also saw the bulk nut and candy section. Now I'm not sure if it was still partially being under the influence of L.S.D., or if the sign really did look so good it may as well have been lit up with flashing neon lights and go-go dancers, "NEW NEON GUMMY WORMS!" Well yeah, at that point, we had to try them. So, like little old ladies in the produce section, casually popping a grape off the bunch to check for freshness and quality, we each popped a bright sugar-coated gummy worm of wonderfulness in our mouths.

Now I can honestly say that they were so good we would've bought at least a pound of them, but before we had the chance to fill up a bag, that same security guard came charging around the corner, so barrel chested even his overrated 1970s' porno mustache was trying to stick its pecs out and flex. "Open your mouths boys!" He demanded.

Still flip-side and thrown into a surreal situation, we failed to even stop chewing, let alone open our mouths. We simply kept gnawing on those delectable gummies like cows chewing their cud. He firmly took each of us by an arm. Me by my left arm with his right hand and my friend by his right arm grasped within the rent-a-cop's left hand and led us to the front of the store. Upon our dubious arrival at the front of the store he promptly paraded us through the only open checkout lane that morning, and right up to the clerk. Like he was stopping an invasion from an evil foreign government, he boasted, "These boys decided to help themselves to a piece of candy in the bulk section."

With a bewildered expression of raised eyebrows, the checkout clerk looks at me, my friend, at his coworker, the grocery bagger, and then directs his glare back at the security guard, "So?" The checkout clerk said in an almost bland and monotone voice, clearly unimpressed with the security guard's supposed big bust. Both of us chuckled a bit, having already realized how overzealous he was being.

"We'll give you a quarter." I stated, trying to bargain.

"Yeah, we're more than willing to pay for them. We were going to buy a pound anyway!" Sonny said, backing me up. Apparently, he had come to the same conclusion I did. New Neon Gummy Worms were too good not to buy and in bulk.

Not getting the praise he felt he deserved, the security guard coldly shut us down. "It's too late for that," he said, as he firmly tugged us to the front of the store, where he made us stand directly in front of the locked plastic cigarette cabinet. "We're going to make an example out of you two."

"Stay here and don't move," he commanded. Still being compliant and honestly still enjoying chawing on our individual new neon gummy worms, we stayed there, looking at the various types and brands of cigarettes, not having been seduced by that hideous dragon yet, we waited for our inevitable fate of being thrust into the local juvenile delinquent programs so many of our friends, peers, and predecessors had already frequented. A few minutes later and nothing but the taste of our neon gummy temptations left, he came back from the manager's office to take us into the office so we could sit and wait for the police. "We're going to make an example out of you two for all of your little shoplifting friends. Make sure you tell them that shoplifting will not be tolerated here." He reiterated with more detail, as if he had busted the biggest and first shoplifting ring in this little American town. FYI, we weren't the biggest, the first, or even a shoplifting ring. Just two teenagers who were in over our heads because of the irresistible temptations of a candied treat and not thinking in the moment.

The manager's office that he led us to was down a longer than necessary hallway. Especially for the size of the office. It was maybe an eight-by-eight-foot room with a warehouse height ceiling, earth-toned color palette, and intimidatingly tall walls. It was like a room from a Tim Burton movie only more color than monochrome. Directly in the line with the southern wall of the office was the door and the manager's desk nestled in the corner, perpendicular off the same wall as the door. Walk through the door and take a quick left, you would've found us. Where my friend and I sat in two identical folding waiting chairs with metal frames and unforgiving metal seats. For the situation, I don't think upholstered seats would've been more comfortable for the very uncomfortable scenario that we were in. The security guard temporarily sat at the manager's desk so he could fill out whatever corporate paperwork that came with catching mastermind criminals like us, to satisfy a corporate machine like that.

But that was where the levity ended. The reality is that I had my personal smoke, a fat quarter ounce of pot (under a full ounce, a misdemeanor at the time), as well as the rest of my personal acid, L.S.D. One count of manslaughter per hit (none of them would be a misdemeanor) on me and my pipe (another minor misdemeanor for paraphernalia). My friend had about the same on him (misdemeanors and manslaughters. None of his manslaughters would've been misdemeanors either).

The situation became even more tense when Sonny tried to conceal his stash by moving it from his pocket to his underwear. For those of you who think this will help you get away with something because it's in that naughty place, and crossing that line would be indignant, or even illegal, think again. Especially if you get locked up on the inside. They will look, and they will find it, because they will look hard and deep. Take that however you like, but know that it's both literal and metaphorical and if they don't find it until you get to jail, guess what? Extra charges for introduction of contraband. The security guard, the only one in the room with us, was busy filling out paperwork and from the looks of it, trying really hard too. So, my friend decided to chance it, and swiftly moved whatever he could from his right pocket to his underwear when he thought the security guard wasn't looking. The security guard snapped his head up and glared at my friend in the same instance that Sonny pulled his now empty hand from his pants. "The cops will find whatever you just tried to hide when they search you."

Sonny snapped right back at him without a second's hesitation, "My dick itched!"

The security guard snickered confidently knowing the police, who would be there shortly, would put us both in place. We spent the rest of what seemed like a lifetime in complete silence. As the security guard finished his paperwork, I was quietly kissing my own ass goodbye. My friend, I imagine, was doing the same. When out of nowhere, Officer Amada and his partner finally walked in.

"Officers!" The overzealous security guard exclaimed, like greeting long lost friends. "I caught these boys shoplifting." He boasted, sounding as if he would get an on-the-spot commendation that he was expecting.

With a disappointing sigh directed at us, Officer Amada gets out his ticket book and with a click of his pen, "What did they try to shoplift and how much was it worth?"

You could almost feel the hot air leave the security guard's over-inflated ego when there was no slap on the back accompanied by a "good one buddy!" From either one of our smalltown cops that showed up. As he choked his disappointment back down, certain that much deserved accommodation must be right around the corner, but business first. "They each ate a gummy worm, and I don't know how much they are worth, individually."

The officers' heads both sank a little lower as Amada let out a different kind of sigh, this time directed at the security guard. "A gummy worm? Really?" He paused for a second, shook his head side-to-side ever so slightly, and begrudgingly continued. "Okay, how much is a gummy worm valued at?"

"I don't know. Twenty-five, fifty cents, maybe? I'm not really sure," replied the security guard with more of his brand of uncertainty.

"We need to know the value, or we can't write them a ticket for shoplifting." Stated Officer Amada, further detailing why.

"Okay. Hold on. I'll find out." said the security officer.

"I'll come with you," said Officer Amada to the security guard. "Stay here, make sure they don't bolt." He tells his partner, who almost followed them, but stops and posts up outside the manager's door, just as he was instructed to. My friend and I waited silently for them to get an individual neon gummy worm from the back of the store, bring it to the front, and weigh it, so they could ascertain the value of our obviously brilliant devious deception perpetrated by members of our elite teenage shoplifting ring.... allegedly (shhh).

It seemed like they had to walk to the back forty acres by the time they got back to the manager's office, in the front of the store. "Ten to fifteen cents each." Officer Amada stated as he walked back into the manager's office and continued to fill out our tickets. We sat silently, waiting in disbelief that we were getting a shoplifting ticket for ten cents let alone that the cops were writing it. We would've offered to pay for them once more, but it would've proven again to be pointless, so we both held our tongues (Don't volunteer information. Don't talk yourself into a deeper hole).

After we both signed our tickets, Officer Amada handed us our copies of the tickets back. They came with, "You boys are free to go." Without hesitation we immediately stood up to leave with a deadened haste, so as to not raise too much suspicion.

"WAIT! You guys aren't going to search 'em?" Exclaimed the security guard, who sounded like a guy who thought he had won a lottery, made a bunch of expensive purchases, and panicked when he found out that he didn't actually win.

"Freeze boys." Calmly but firmly said Officer Amada. Being ever compliant, so as not to make things worse, we did (Never run. Do as you are instructed). But like young bucks caught in headlights, on a dangerous mountain road, in the middle of the night, where we had jumped down from a small cliff, and there is nowhere else to go but into the grill of that big rig semi or off the other side of the mountain road, down another cliff. "You didn't search them?" Calmly and even more disappointingly, with a side order of judgement, asked Officer Amada, looking at the grocery store security officer with both eyebrows raised.

I thought, "Damn, almost got away," as the paper blotter acid in my pocket instantly felt heavier and hotter as if turning to molten lead. I'm sure my friend had similar feelings of doom and demise.

"I was waiting for you guys!" Exclaimed the security guard. Replying with throwing his arms in the air, gesturing towards the officer, flailing his arms about to try and help him explain his actions in a desperate and animated flirtation with his justification.

Officer Amada calmly turned and looked at the two of us and again said, "You boys are free to go." And as calmly as possible we turned and walked away, until we were out of sight. Although I imagine it must have looked like fireworks that were trying not to explode. It sure felt that way. The same way a person with the sudden urgency of diarrhea tries to get to the nearest toilet as quickly possible, before anything worse happens. As soon as we were certain that we were out of sight, it was a mad dash to my red 1986 Toyota Corolla and out of their parking lot as fast as possible. Olympic sprinters would've been proud. Even the ones who have blades on their legs, and we still managed to not shoot any cute blonds, imagine that.

In case you forgot, or perhaps you are on the edge of your seat with anticipation, what was that sage advice we received? When our day in court came around it was in a makeshift courtroom, as the traditional courtroom was under renovation. I had even attended a religious service in the same room by an up-and-coming church that leased the space on Sundays as they lacked a building to call their own place of worship at the time. It was one of the older buildings in town. Most likely constructed in the heydays of the old west. As such, the wood paneled walls of the room were lined with a matching handmade chair rail about three feet off the carpeted floor, encircling the entire room. They had a portable wooden banister that separated court personnel from those summoned and the lawyers. And a turn of the century tin tile ceiling above it all. The judge and the recorder sat on a slightly elevated platform behind another banister. With the bailiff standing guard on this side of the banister and all the way to the right of the room. Our cases were called simultaneously, "The people versus Grant Kinion and the people versus Sonny Vale. Please step forward." We respectfully complied, and the two of us gathered at the defendant's table. As we were both under eighteen, we had to be accompanied by a guardian. Each of our mothers filled that role by coming with us, but they stayed seated in the middle of the courtroom, next to each other in the unforgiving metal folding chairs that were put out before everyday court was in session and picked up every day after court was adjourned.

In our small town, that was Tuesdays and Thursdays for city court and we had but two city judges. The judge presiding over our case was Judge Hitchell. The judge spoke to us a bit, first with the usual questions for juveniles. Off handed questions that allude to family situations, financial, and living status, etc. Checking for signs of abuse, intelligence, and poverty level. And then....

"Are you boys both still in school?" Judge Hitchell asked.

"Yes sir." We both replied, one at a time, and in an orderly fashion.

"What kind of grades can you maintain while on juvenile probation?" He asked us each, first my friend. "Mr. Vale? We will start with you."

"All As" Sonny replied.

"And Mr. Kinion?"

"All Bs" I answered, with the intent of not wanting to put in as much work as my friend.

The judge looks up from his files and laptop screen, his eyebrows leading his eyes towards us with more than just a glance for the first time since he called our cases up. His head still slightly tilted downward, staring at us from over the top of his glasses, eyebrows still raised like two grizzlies standing tall, intimidatingly gauging its prey. "You two, approach the bench." He turns and looks in the direction of his recorder. "This will be off record." As we promptly and humbly approached the front of the courtroom, we both noticed the recorder moving her hands from the keyboard to her lap. We both leaned closer, hugging the wooden banister of separation between the judge and the soon to be judged. He pushed the microphone aside, so it was completely off record as well as private. The rest of the courtroom couldn't hear him tell us, "You boys are a lot smarter than most of the young men who come through my courtroom." He leans in closer to keep his next words even further confidential in the small but crowded courtroom, his eyebrows still arched, but this time more like a wise old owl giving advice (on something more than how many licks does it take to get to the center of a…well, never mind). Almost magnetically, we do the same and to get even closer as well, leaning over the banister a bit further without technically crossing the border it represented. Our hearing was only slightly restricted by the distance created by the banister still separating us and the recorder in front of the judge, yet still far from an earshot of the rest of the courtroom. He continued in an even lower private tone. "So, if you're going to be blowing a lot of dope…DON'T. GET. CAUGHT." In a firm yet profound whisper.

For two young adult teenagers, what he said could not have been more profound. It was like that scene in the movie Field of Dreams, only our guiding advice wasn't a whisper from a mysterious breeze, but quiet advice from an administrator of The Constitution. DON'T GET CAUGHT! Of course! So simple, yet so profound, and so obvious once we heard it. It was kind of like we couldn't believe we hadn't thought of it ourselves before now and felt a little stupid for not. At the same time, it seemed so powerful, we felt like we had the keys to the universe, or at least the key to successful drug use. The quintessential, "How to Get Away with It." DON'T-GET-CAUGHT. Meaning keep your head down. Especially don't break little laws if you're breaking bigger ones. So many different interpretations of such a new and profound thought. That now seemed like a keystone for our lives. And yet, it seemed so simple. Again, it was like, "Why didn't we think of that?" Because we probably should have.

Even though what we did wasn't technically shoplifting, but rather called "grazing," it was also done unconsciously. If we had just loaded up a bag of them and taken them up front with our donuts we intended to buy, instead of taste testing them, we wouldn't have had a problem. But we also wouldn't have had a problem if we were silver haired old ladies, and it was a grape off a bunch, as that security guard wasn't ever interested in following little old ladies.

Furthermore, if we had taken what we had on us out of our pockets and left the "elicits" in the car in the parking lot, we wouldn't have had those worries and potentially much larger problems in the store. Even though we managed to avoid worse charges by God gracing us, like Neo in the Matrix dodging bullets. If we had left the stuff that was on us in the car, we would've had to remember to put those things back on us when we got back in the car, in case we got pulled over. So, even better would have been to leave what we had on us at the house, stashed safely. After all, if you're going to the store to get groceries of any kind, but donuts especially, you're typically going right back home or to work. No need to get high, so you don't need to carry your supply. Lessening risk by eliminating unnecessary risk. From that moment on, I can say that I planned ahead a lot more and I took better care when taking inventory of myself and my vehicle, which I did a lot more from that point on. Many-a-slip between a cup and a lip, doesn't mean you don't do everything in your power to prevent it. It means shit happens, sometimes it is unexpected and unpreventable, except for the times that it is preventable. But you should know, it is still always best to not sip shit.

Rule Ten: Every Action Has a Reaction

Drug abuse, whether legal like alcohol, tobacco, and prescription medications, or recreational, illegal drug use, including the latest greatest thing that hasn't become illegal yet is not a fairy tale story. It never is. Drug abuse has severe, and sometimes deadly, consequences and you will lose. It may be employment, family, friends, freedoms, health, home, love, life, lucidity, memories, maturity, money, and the list goes on. The more severe the reaction is, the more you need to realize you should do less, or even none at all of that particular substance, and honestly there are people who shouldn't do any substances whatsoever. And there are substances themselves that should also never be done. Not everything that can be consumed should.

Currently, more, and more, people are beginning to wake up to the medical potential of certain "street" drugs, marijuana, first and foremost. Drugs that are seemingly turning over a new leaf. Drugs that have had a bad reputation, similar to a reformed ex-convict. Drugs that have turned legal in some areas and are starting to turn licit in others. And people are even realizing that recreational use is not only okay with some of these alleged "street drugs," but they can be way less harmful in the long run than some of the already legal recreational substances. That's right, I called nicotine, alcohol, even caffeine, and others, recreational substances. In a day and age when even caffeine has been modified, compounded, and combined with vitamins, minerals, and herbs, so much so that it is now giving some people heart attacks, yeah, substances.

It is important to have a realistic perspective, along with a guide. A guide that essentially says, "This is what you should experience, this is what to watch out for, this is what to avoid." This guide is for the beginners and the advanced drug users alike. It is as well for the medical provider and patient, as well as the curious, who don't necessarily want to partake but need, or desire, a deeper understanding. It is to help navigate, understand, and fly straight in a field that like everything else, has the potential to be taken way too far and in this instance, already misunderstood and misused on epic proportions. It is to help you watch out for the potential of abuse. So, this is my forte and my experience used to help as many as possible. Yours will be more unique than different, but this is basically what you're going for and looking out for. This book is how to learn how to handle "it" and how to "maintain" with "moderation" and human decency.

If you still don't understand why someone would want to take the risk of addiction, legal troubles, and even death to do drugs, I will tell you again. Drugs are really fucking fun and enjoyable. If you already do drugs, or are curious about drugs, know what you're risking. Your life, your freedom, your sanity, and your health. For most reasonable people that is enough reason to not even take the chance. But you should know it's also because you have no idea how much fun drugs can be, or how necessary relief is and how much it can be a need to have even a temporary reprieve from debilitating ailments.

When it comes to prescription medications that are addictive, understand that if they weren't at least enjoyable on some level, they wouldn't be addictive. If they weren't helpful and absolutely necessary for a large number of patients, they wouldn't be legal, albeit restricted and highly regulated for good reasons. And if you're a medical provider, that is the first thing you need to understand and explain to your patients. You need to explain why people get addicted. Honesty is always the best policy. You want to make sure that your patients know that if this is for an acute temporary situation, that these medications are, in most situations, exactly that, temporary. If it is not a temporary situation but turns into a quality-of-life situation, these medications need to be used in a way that is sparingly, as it is potent and effective beyond when your body builds a tolerance for the intoxication part. You need to explain what an addict feels like when they have that draw, that undeniable pull, that makes it harder, and harder, for an addict to say no. And you need to show that to them by having them take yearly, or even bi-yearly, sabbaticals. At least for a while, so they can see that when they developed a tolerance, and it wasn't getting them totally wasted like it did in the beginning, it was still greatly reducing their pain, their anxiety, their ailments. They need to know at that point, whatever relief they can achieve, is as good as it gets, and they need to be able to accept that, so they don't "chase the dragon." And you need to explain to them how to watch themselves for any sign of the psychological and/or the chemically induced magnetic pull that is addiction. You need to explain that with opioid painkillers they want it to abate eighty to ninety percent of their chronic pain, not all of it. This is so the patient is still aware of their physical limitations. To keep from aggravating their existing conditions, making things worse, because they can't accurately gauge their pain level.

Now that I have explained those experiences to everyone, you don't have to experience them yourselves. I've told you what your patients will experience, and what they don't want to experience, which is what they need to watch out for more than you, the medical provider. The responsibility for taking these medications needs to be put back with the patient. Otherwise, it's too easy for a medical provider to violate, innocent until proven guilty, and jump right into assumed guilt.

The best thing the FDA/CDC has done in a long time (maybe ever) is come up with the Morphine Scale. When the FDA and CDC originally sounded the war horn on the opioid crisis they encouraged as many people to get taken off as many pain medications as possible. People didn't like that. For those who are legitimate patients, it wasn't being cut off from their medication as much as it was being made to suffer needlessly by people who have zero proper firsthand perspective into the situation. At that point a lot of patients refused to suffer, or didn't want to, or simply couldn't anymore. Some self-medicated with alcohol or street drugs and sometimes both. And hence patients started going to jail, accidentally overdosing on unreliable street drugs, drinking themselves to death, or committed suicide. The FDA and CDC pretty much came out and said, "We may have overreacted. Turns out it is better to prescribe these medications, and help patients deal with their pain, than it is to expect them to just deal with it on their own. Which has led to patients self-medicating in a Russian Roulette sort of way." I'm adlibbing once more, but because of that to-and-fro, that back-and-forth from the government, now even medical providers are afraid to prescribe them. Hence, coming out with The Morphine Scale. The scale that equates all opioid pain medication to morphine. If you score too high on the scale, you need to be watched like a hawk for addiction, cut down on dosage, or even cut off entirely. Score low enough, and you are at no, or low risk for addiction. But here is the deal, if a medical patient who is chronic or permanently disabled, has very little joy or happiness in their life, how much should an addiction or the potential for developing an addiction be counted as an important factor? As a matter of fact, being disabled is pretty damn miserable and depressing, despite the brave front some of us put on. Not to mention the unrealistically jovial demeanor people portraying patients on prescription advertisements act. Is an addiction really a major factor when it can give momentary happiness and relief, that otherwise is nonexistent? Especially if getting high occasionally keeps someone from taking their own life. If you're dying, or in your eighties or nineties, does it matter if you are starting to become addicted, have been addicted for a long time, or are addicted? Or should it matter more that you're as comfortable as possible? I promise that when someone passes away, they cut themselves off with no additional suffering than was necessary. As little pain as possible and no withdrawal symptoms. And without professional help, imagine that. But especially when a medical provider cuts that seventy-, eighty-, or ninety-year-old off from their addictive medication and force them to go through chemical withdrawals, you are making an elderly person suffer for no reason, simply out of ignorance, and for your own ego, and solely out of concern for covering your own ass. In that instance you hurt someone, you didn't help them. You only helped yourself. I would argue that it does hurt even you, the provider, in the long run, as there is such a thing as spiritual currency.

How to Smoke Marijuana

Understand that absolutely everyone has cannabinoid receptors. You, me, even the fragile eighty-eight-year-old grandmother that lives a few dwellings down from you and has never even known anyone who smoked pot, let alone attempted to consume it herself. For those not in the know, cannabis is the scientific term for marijuana. Thus, cannabinoid receptors receive what makes pot, well pot. Mainly THC, but also CBD, CBC (and a whole shit ton of others) and along with terpene profiles, all allow us to benefit from its many medicinal properties and yes, the THC specifically lets us also get high from it. It specifically enables it to be intoxicating and what people have come to call "Stoned."

When you first begin to use marijuana, or rather the first time you use it, the experience can be very intense, even overwhelming, and off-putting for some. Especially these days when it is so much more potent than it was in the 1990s, and exponentially more so than 1960's quintessential hippy weed. If you do find it overwhelming or way too intense, rest assured this is temporary and not how it is on a permanent basis. Only the first few times with emphasis on the first time. If you did happen to enjoy how intense it was at first, know that you will never achieve this super heightened sensitive state again. That usually is only the first time. Don't seek that out either. If you seek that first initial high that you had with any drug or medication, you are essentially "chasing the dragon" (only with something other than heroin) and blowing right over moderation, which will lead to problems down the road. The adjustment period for marijuana is reasonably short. Especially when you consider that most antidepressants take four to six weeks to determine if they work. If they don't, the safe way is to wean off of them to discontinue. Another four to six weeks after that, you're ready to try another brain chemical altering antidepressant which you will know if it works or not a typical four to six weeks later. And if that one doesn't, well you get the idea. It's a vicious cycle.

Use very little marijuana to begin with. Especially when you use it medicinally. The goal of using it as medication is to achieve the best potential outcome while getting complete ailment control or as close as possible, while using the smallest amount possible. Less is more, the same methodology that should be used with most everything in life, but especially with prescription medications and recreational substances alike. And only intentionally use marijuana in excess to achieve the same effect you would get from an anxiety cessation medication a.k.a. barbiturates, like Xanax or Ativan or Valium, but again only when needed. Or in excess when you need the same relief for a migraine cessation. Only in the case of marijuana, you're not limited on dosage, you don't need to wait an hour or two for it to kick in and see if it did or didn't work, you can't overdose on it, and it takes minutes for each dose (or in this case each hit) to take effect, which usually means close to instant relief. That also means you consume it until you feel relief from a migraine. Not, if the second dose of medication doesn't work, like in the case of Maxalt, you're absolutely screwed.

The goal when using marijuana recreationally is to get high without ruining your life, in any aspect. Similar to how some people come home at night and have a glass of wine, beer, or a stiff drink to unwind. They aren't necessarily alcoholics, simply because they don't abuse it or take it to that unreasonable level where people act unreasonably almost by default. You don't let a substance control you. If it reaches the point where any substance does have more control than you do, you have reached the point of failure. Time to check yourself. When it comes to recreational drug use, marijuana should be used as an experience enhancer, not as an experience only. Although, until you get a little tolerance and experience with it, it will be an experience all on its own. Don't remain in that state. After the initial, very intense, adjustment period, especially these days because marijuana is so much stronger than it was when it was illegal, enjoy it.

Whether you're medical, recreation, or both, you will have a good time. And please, have a good time, it is meant to be enjoyed. That should be the number one goal of any form of intoxication (spiritual applications both included and excluded), but for now I'm encouraging you to enjoy the process. You'll be able to laugh; no, you will laugh at things that normally wouldn't be as funny without being stoned. As it will help you relax and drop your guard a little, if you wish it. You most probably have heard it before, "laughter is the best medicine." Well, you will giggle like a giddy little girl. You will be happy. Maybe happier than ever before, but at least more jovial than you have been in a long time. And when you eat, whatever you eat, it will be the best tasting thing you have ever put in your mouth. Full disclosure, don't try to eat something that already tastes bad and expect it to taste good. Marijuana is great and good and fun, but it is not that great. It is, however, great enough that you will see things as you have never seen them before. A fresh perspective with new eyes. You will have epiphanies that you otherwise wouldn't. And you'll be able to understand and bond with someone on a whole different level, that was unavailable before.

The first time I smoked marijuana was with my oldest friend, Sonny. Sonny lived in what appeared to be an affluent house until you learned that he and his family lived in such a nice house at the unfortunate expense of his older brother's health. Connor, Sonny's older brother, was born normal with good health, that many of us are fortunate enough to be granted with, but he had that particular blood type that doesn't jive with vaccines. If you aren't someone who has this blood type, or you don't know anyone who has that blood type, they can't have vaccinations. Messes them up. His doctors had this knowledge, they knew what it would do to him, and they gave him the newborn vaccinations that most of us get anyway. It took him from a healthy newborn baby boy with every bit as bright of a future as the rest of us, to one with cerebral palsy, epilepsy, at the highest levels of severity of being physically and mentally developmentally disabled, also accompanied by an inability to speak. Just one example to touch on how dangerous drugs are, and how dangerous all drugs, including medications, have the potential to be.

One of the current prohibitionist misconceptions is that marijuana causes anxiety. The misconception comes from two different misconceptions. Newbies who are beginning to smoke marijuana with no guidance or expectation of what is going to happen. This is actually one of those learning curves to doing drugs, but specifically with pot. Marijuana will initially cause a paranoia sensation, but I will argue that it is simply a part of being in a new headspace and learning your surroundings. Similar to dropping an animal into a new environment. It's going to take a bit for that animal to become orientated and not be on high alert all the time. If you're paranoid, or think you are, you have anxiety. Anxiety of the unknown, and if I'm bluntly honest, in this case and arguably others, the fear of nothing. It takes some time to realize that you are letting yourself be paranoid. That's why it helps to have someone who is experienced with you to help guide you through it, that you can trust. That is someone you can trust, not necessarily someone you want to trust.

Someone who will say, "You're just high, don't let it make you paranoid. Enjoy the ride." And then demonstrates exactly that. If you're doing it medically, (after you get the basics down or as the label says on medications with the potential for an intoxicated state, "DO NOT DRIVE OR OPERATE VEHICLES OR HEAVY MACHINERY UNTIL YOU KNOW HOW THIS MEDICATION WILL AFFECT YOU" or "MAY CAUSE DROWSINESS") consume slowly until your ailments are under control, then enjoy the ride of the high. But still, don't drive. It is still illegal to operate a vehicle under the influence of anything, no matter how adjusted you are or become. This is where marijuana rules and most prescription chemicals suck. Marijuana is not addictive, nor can you overdose on it. For most medications, overdosing is not only a possibility, but either means death or a profoundly worse life by many various means. So, if you feel like shit because of one, two, or more ailments and marijuana helps you feel a whole lot better to the point that you are able to enjoy life, and laugh a little (or a lot), have at it, enjoy, indulge. At that point you're not getting high, you're taking medication to mitigate life altering ailments. This is called "achieving quality of life." And the second cause of anxiety is from people overusing marijuana and marijuana concentrates. Again, moderation in all things.

Why would you take one medication for each ailment, and at least one more medication for at least one of the side effects of those medications, and possibly more medications to mitigate the side effects from the additional medications or from the combinations, and however many more medications for those additional side effects? When you can take one herbal medication that not only handles multiple symptoms, but once you become adjusted to it, you will find out that it is far less intoxicating than most chemical-based prescription medication, and with none of the life altering side effects.

If you are taking marijuana recreationally, again it is not addictive, on any level. Indulge, enjoy, but don't let it interfere with your life. Don't dismiss life's chores to get high. Don't smoke and drive. It's the same as not drinking and driving. And for those who are well versed with Mary Jane, I get it. Marijuana can be, and usually is, an entirely different level of intoxication than alcohol. People who don't smoke, but do drink, do not understand that contrast either. So don't be the few who ruin it for the rest of us because you view it as unfair, it's not. It will, however, eventually all come into focus, be patient. Don't go to work or appointments reeking of pot (especially court dates). It will affect your performance and hence the outcome. If you have a marijuana leaf Hawaiian shirt, pot leaf tattoos, miller lite hat, you will get searched, and you will get a sobriety/dui check anytime you see the police. If you dress gung-ho enough, you will get searched more. It does not matter that profiling is illegal. It works, and law enforcement on most levels cannot do their jobs or protect and serve without it. Think that profiling is wrong, all you want. It is probable cause that has been shunned under false pretenses. And arguing otherwise is like arguing that traffic cops using speed traps or unmarked vehicles is cheating and unfair. Only to those who want to get away with something and end up getting caught anyway. And if you're the person constantly pulling the shades apart to look outside, someone will eventually notice. If it's the wrong person, you will give yourself away. As in, if you look paranoid, you probably are for a reason, which puts you on the radar. I'm telling you right now, we are coming upon a time in human history that will hold everyone accountable as everything that can be taken too far, has been taken too far. The only way to still fly under the radar is to not be seen, or heard, so no one speaks of it.

I was never comfortable with smoking and driving. Some of the people I knew, not so much. To them it was as casual as smoking a cigarette while driving. One day I was going snowboarding with my childhood best friend and his older cousin, let's call him Blanche. Blanche was driving us to Telluride in his new shiny work truck. Blanche rolls and lights a joint (while simultaneously being behind the wheel) and we begin to pass it around the cab of his truck. At one of the few intersections on our rural journey, I had the joint but there were other vehicles around so I had it down and out of sight until I could hit it, out of the eye shot of prying eyes. It was a day and age when cell phones weren't quite so popular that everybody had one, but popular enough that you also never knew who did have one, better safe than sorry. As I held it below the precipice of the passenger window. Blanche, becoming impatient (a sign that you're out of control and putting too much value on getting high) exclaimed angrily, "Hit that shit and pass it!"

My best friend, sitting in the backseat of the truck cab, knew full well that what I was doing was right, and Blanche was being an impatient fiend. So, Sonny spoke up, "Yeah Grant, just look right at them and point to the magnetic business sign on the door while you take a big ass hit."

That let the air right out of his pompous ass. "Oh, I forgot about that." Blanche said with the kind of humility that comes with being shown you're the ass, with couth. Again, don't advertise. If you don't want to get busted and you don't want to cause problems, because the name of the game is getting high, it is not, make it harder to get high. Then don't be that guy, don't be a Blanche.

As previously mentioned, when you do have enough experience, whether that means you have a reasonable amount of tolerance or not, a good rule of thumb with marijuana is when you smoke, only take a small portion of the greens, by using as little fire as possible, so each hit tastes optimally good. Whether in a group or smoking marijuana alone, in both a recreation or medical setting, this method will make your marijuana stretch way further and thus you get more use out of a smaller amount, making it go further, both in longevity and potency of the high you or your group can obtain. Versus everyone taking the biggest hit with the most amount of flame as possible, a.k.a. "scavenger hits," which also leaves harsh feelings. Etiquette is important, especially for those who practice it. If you don't think etiquette is important, consider how you feel when someone is polite versus rude, or even how you feel when someone selfishly takes advantage of you. That all could've been avoided with a little etiquette and common courtesy.

Anywhere from about the eighth to the twentieth time you smoke marijuana, your cannabinoid receptors open all the way up and your tolerance gets to a level where you can maintain a small amount. This is where you begin to be able to keep up in a conversation. It is where you don't lose track of the task at hand, or the subject of discussion, because you're high. Or at least you're not losing track all the time. And this is when your memory starts to be affected profoundly less, and less. And all of that will improve even more, down the road, with continued use. When you truly get the hang of maintaining, marijuana can become a genuine experience enhancer, as well as one of the most useful medications you may ever need. I hope you don't need medication of any kind, but if you do, this is where marijuana has the most benefits for a marijuana utilizing medical patient like me, and even reasonable medical benefits for a recreational user, like the mass majority of other people who smoke pot.

Don't get me wrong, marijuana can be abused, like everything and anything. It is one of the main reasons I'm writing this book. If you don't abuse it, you won't lose it, and people won't misunderstand it. When someone smokes so much that they forget appointments, ignore their responsibilities, or they can't even keep up with the conversation in their head, let alone keep up in a conversation with another person, or even have a polite one. That is when you end up doing things unsafely, and you start to appear unintelligent. Or if you pass out from over consumption, it makes you look glutenous and lethargic. This is where society says, "See, pot is bad," simply from observing one or two people who over indulged. I can tell you there are multitudes of medical patients who do (or would do) far better on it than without. However, due to still existing prejudices, stereotypes, misunderstandings, and miseducation about it, there are still far too many people who remain over-medicated, while simultaneously being under-treated, and still over-intoxicated by way of being over medicated and made to suffer far more than they ever should. When they could instead smoke a little pot and be way more themselves with way less suffering, while taking fewer medications, and becoming less intoxicated. The conspiracy theorist in my head says it is all in the name of profit for the pharmaceutical and medical companies. They see more money in treating rather than curing. The rational side of me says, I'm not that far off. But, in an optimal world, if everyone is at peak health, won't we all prosper and profit far beyond a sandbagging approach to monetizing healthcare, instead of progressing it.

My Specific Medical Marijuana Uses

Keep in mind, I'm not a doctor. I'm a human being who has suffered greatly. Not only because of the accumulation of my many injuries and accidents, which led me into the hands of the medical field, but I have also suffered greatly at the hands of the medical field, and its medications, until I finally realized that I needed to figure some things out for myself. Learning to listen to my own body is and was paramount and every bit as important, if not more so, than listening to my medical provider. So, take my advice for what it's worth, and find what works for you. Use the ten rules in this book as guidelines. And you may come up with some more from your own experiences. This is what I have experienced and observed with responsible medicinal marijuana use.

One of the great things about marijuana that trumps the various chemical prescription medications that individually can treat one or two ailments, out of the many ailments that marijuana can treat by itself, there is no thirty-to-ninety-minute wait time. Let alone a for-to-six-week build-up in your system, results are nearly instant. So, take a hit, give it a minute, take another, give it a minute, and repeat until you get your desired relief. If you need higher doses of marijuana quicker, take your hits in quicker succession or even power hit it, but only if you're desperate and etiquette isn't required. That's another great thing about traditional marijuana over prescription medications, good luck overdosing on it. Whereas if you reach a limit with certain medications and your pain, or anxiety, or anything else for that matter isn't relieved at all or enough, you can suffer or take a chance. For medical marijuana, until you have the hang of it, use it when you must, use it when you need to. If regimented use of marijuana is what you need, then do a regiment. No one wants you to suffer, and that is exactly what marijuana is useful for on a practical medical level, helping to ease your suffering. Once you do have your legs under you, here is my dosage for what ails me. Again, I am not a medical professional. I am a patient who got fed up with people telling me a chemically induced walking dead coma was the best I could hope for and that I really was better off, I just didn't realize it. Well, I found a better way, and these are my personal observations.

For migraines, smoke until the migraine is gone, or you're tired enough from being stoned that you can try and sleep through it. This is one of those situations where the earlier you catch an encroaching migraine and try to treat it, the better. Otherwise, a small regiment of a few hits, three to seven days a week, depending on the severity and frequency of your migraines, should work well as a migraine preventative. If you have migraines as severe as mine, smoke. Being stoned a little or a lot is one million times better than suffering from a migraine, which is excruciating, and in my opinion, one of the most painful experiences anyone can have.

If you have anxiety, again, less is more. The trick here is to consume enough to take the edge off, until your anxiety isn't unbearable. Smoke too much or consume a too potent source of THC (concentrates), and you might make your anxiety worse. If your tolerance is too high, it makes managing anxiety with marijuana more difficult, especially if you are having an extreme anxiety attack. This one takes some practice, and as I mentioned, is easier managed with a low tolerance level. Remember the learning curve I spoke of? If you can't take anxiety medications or their lesser known, and not-so-widely accepted, herbal counterparts for any reason, then marijuana can be a wonderful alternative. It's right in the middle of prescriptions, herbs, and

OTCs in a vin diagram. Marijuana is a "one stone, many birds," kind of treatment, as it is versatile beyond any of the three groups separately, with very few side effects compared to the other three groups individually. The trick of treating anxiety attacks with marijuana is to keep your marijuana tolerance as low as possible. You can do this by taking periodical sabbaticals to lower your tolerance as needed, or as often as possible. If your tolerance remains super low, the success rate of treating anxiety attacks with marijuana increases exponentially. As it does with treating anything else.

If you have an appetite problem and you need to eat for health reasons, but you can't because you're nauseated, or you have an eating disorder, marijuana can work great for this. It's called, "The Munchies," and they are at their strongest in the middle to tail end of the high. Consume enough to be happy and satisfied (both marijuana and food), but beware. It really is easy to overeat when you're high because everything tastes so much better. Well, almost everything. Always remember, making chicken salad out of chicken shit is only an expression. There are some things, like chicken shit, that should never be consumed and won't taste good no matter how much weed you smoke. In other words, if you don't like the taste of beets, for example, or you dislike the taste of anything else for that matter, "The Munchies" most likely won't change that.

If you have a nausea problem (and you're not pregnant), smoke until your nausea is relieved. It will happen much quicker than you think, as long as your nausea doesn't come from a virus or bacteria. In the case of getting and being sick, use marijuana for relief and ease of your various ailments, if you can. Know that abusing marijuana can cause you to be sicker than you have ever been, so again, less is more. This is also where extracts/concentrates are not so wonderful. It's great to get really high on very little, but extracts can sometimes make something that is very useful, like THC, and turn it into something that is sometimes too potent and that can be counterproductive.

If you have insomnia, or you have a problem going to sleep, try to smoke before bedtime. You have two options here for using marijuana for going to sleep. You can either smoke until you are ready to pass out, or you can plan it so the tail end of your high is at your bedtime. It's simply the natural process of getting high with marijuana. First you get high and feel really good for a while, when you start to come down, or a little bit before, is when your munchies will be the strongest, followed by, hopefully getting tired enough that you want to go to sleep. I will say this effect was more profound with what would've been considered mid-grade and low-grade marijuana back in the 1990s. But use whatever method of the two works for you at the time.

If your problem is staying asleep, whether you also wake from pain, like me, or for other reasons, and you can't simply go back to sleep, you can do what is called a "wake and bake." It is quite literal. You will want to load a bowl, roll a joint, ready your vaporizer, or whatever your preferred method is, the night before. That way it is ready as soon as you wake up. If you wake up because of bladder or bowel problems, consider keeping it in the bathroom so you can smoke as you do your business. I know, for most of us, it sounds a step shy of eating a hoagie while cutting a loaf on the throne, but when you have a medical necessity, you do what you gotta do. The idea with a "wake and bake" is to smoke right away, when you first wake up, so that you don't completely wake all the way up. From there, it helps you pass back out promptly, and hopefully for a long time, or at least as long as possible. There have been times in my life before marijuana became so readily available because of legalization, when my pain and other various ailments have only allowed me fifteen minutes of sleep every couple of days. And times when I'd go up to four days at a time without any sleep at all, another bonus from my physical pain and migraines. So, do what you need to sleep with marijuana's assistance. It's safe and can't be fatally abused like sleep aids, tranquilizers, self-medicating with alcohol, or anything else that has the potential to knock you out. This next part is important.... Make sure you smoke in a location and fashion that you won't accidentally start a fire. That's why I recommend a bowl. Don't clean it out until morning. Let the pot or ashes kick it in the bowl. Simply tamp the smoldering weed out gently until the embers, a.k.a. the cherry has been snuffed out. The main goal with a wake and bake is to go back to sleep. The secondary goal, however equally important, is not to start a fire, because your priority is getting more of some much needed sleep, not burning down your dwelling.

If you have a problem with constipation and a stool softener or laxative feel like they cause a volatile reaction, try some weed. Smoking pot can not only help to relieve constipation but in some cases, it can have the potential to promote bowel movements. As long as I haven't been constipated for days, usually due to taking additional medications outside of my regiment, smoking a little marijuana is a kinder alternative to medications that have side effects that mimic the flu. Keep in mind, this may not work for severe constipation, but if it does, what a relief that would be.

I will tell you that if you are an individual in need of additional pain management and your painkillers don't quite get the job done, add a few hits of pot. It will have a compounding effect for increasing the amount of pain that is mitigated, while not increasing your chances of overdosing like taking an additional prescription pill(s) would. Marijuana, when used medically, should be used like any other drug. Less is more, as long as you use enough. And it's more like herbal supplements in terms of possible side effects, few and far between, but proceed with caution. The side effects of marijuana are getting tired, increased appetite, uncontrollable and random laughter with fits of happiness, and if you're smoking it, a possible cough. You can become a little paranoid, but again, this is a beginner/lightweight thing. Paranoia will go away as your body and mind adjust to accepting marijuana. And as far as short-term memory loss is concerned, that too will improve and eventually won't be a factor at all. I question slowed reflexes, as there are athletes that have won the Olympics while having marijuana in their system, so take that one with a grain of salt. For the most part, you should know there are health consequences for smoking anything that produces any kind of tar, or in the case of marijuana, it's called resin. And there are almost always consequences for using or doing anything in excess, which is why I encourage extreme caution with marijuana extracts and concentrates. Know if you do choose to consume marijuana edibles, that method does take thirty to sixty minutes to take effect and even though the intoxication from edibles is usually a lesser high than smoking it, you are still imbibing a concentrate and thus it may have unintended adverse reactions.

I will also tell you that even though I have neurological ailments that mimic seizures, they are not. As such a CBD or CBC based tincture doesn't help me, but that doesn't mean that it definitively won't help you. The neat thing about CBD/CBC based medications is they come from the hemp plant, not the marijuana plant. Distant cousins sure, but hemp cannot get you high as it lacks THC in an adequate amount. So, if that is one of the things that has been stopping you from trying a hemp-based tincture for your seizures, it's not an actual thing. Try it, it might change your life for the better.

The Pitfalls of Prescriptions

I replaced more than a few medications with marijuana. Medicinal marijuana if you want to get specific. What's the difference? I would love to tell you that recreational marijuana and recreational marijuana products are for enjoyment purposes only. And medical marijuana helps you cope with as many ailments as possible while having the least number of drawbacks as possible. But the reality is, they are interchangeable. The idea that they are separate only exists in the letter of the law and arbitrary regulations. But the idea that marijuana can replace many medications as a safer and better alternative is absolutely grounded in reality and in no way limited to the valid uses myself and many others have already discovered.

For starters, I was taking Phenergan for nausea, as well as Maxalt or Imitrex for migraine abortion. And if you're offended that I used the word "abortion" to refer to getting rid of something as horrible as a migraine, like me at one time, you have never had a migraine. Don't look for things to be offended by, and you won't feel offended all the time. I also replaced Ativan/Lorazepam (a benzodiazepine) for anxiety attacks, Lunesta/Tylenol PM/and many other sleep aids, over the counter, and prescription. An appetite-increasing medication…just kidding, there isn't a safe prescription for that. I needed a migraine prevention medication, that also didn't exist in a traditional from-the-doctor prescription, only in off-label use medications, when my medical trials began, but they claim to manufacture a few now. Most claim they can take your migraine days and cut them in half. In my case, that would take my twenty-four to thirty migraines a month down to twelve to fifteen migraines in a month. A significant improvement, no doubt. Until you realize that with proper use of medical marijuana, I have taken my twenty-four to thirty severe migraines every month down to seven in the last fifteen years since medical marijuana has been legal in Colorado. That's about one migraine every two years or twenty-four months, that I have not been able to prevent or abort. Let's say I was able to take one of the new migraine prevention medications that weren't even out fifteen years ago. It means that, in the best-case scenario, I would have experienced two-hundred-eighty-eight to three-hundred-sixty-five migraines every two years, instead of the one migraine every two years with the assistance of medical marijuana. To be fair, and full disclosure, so no one can accuse me of manipulating the numbers, that's on average. Still, keep in mind, not all solutions will work for all people.

The combined side effects of a nausea medication, a migraine medication, a sleep aid medication, an anxiety medication, even though not all are taken at the same time, but taken throughout the day, still had this brutal combined intoxicated effect. Especially on top of my more than necessary painkiller and muscle relaxer, that is the kind of high that makes you look like a zombie from an outsider's perspective, and in the best-case scenario, on autopilot from your perspective. And once more, it was a level of high a street junkie would be jealous of. So why take all of those chemicals and end up grumpy and irritable after a time period of being so worthlessly high you don't remember a fair amount of it, if you remember any of it at all, when you can smoke a little pot and eventually remain functional without full blown ailments, after you become adjusted to it? Versus ending up being a pharmaceutical junkie via doctor's orders, or street junkie by way of an unintentional addiction when you are only trying to self-medicate to feel better. Or an even worse reasoning when becoming addicted, because you wanted to get a little higher?

What you should be thinking is, "is any addiction intentional?" If you try coke, or meth, or heroin, or fentanyl, and you end up getting addicted, which odds say if you try it, you will get addicted and I was an anomaly, is that an intentional addiction? You just wanted to get high. Who actually knew how strong that particular pull, from that particular substance, would be for you? A certain, particular person in your own rights. But you knew the risks, didn't you?

Own it. You might not have known the extent of what it meant to be addicted, to be hooked on a hardcore street drug, but you did know it was a one way path for most people, and whether you convinced yourself you would win a lottery that doesn't exist, of being above human psychology and chemical addiction, or whatever rationalization you used, you rolled the dice and came up short. That's why they call it "shooting craps." If that's the case, please seek professional help. If you can't be happy with being reasonably stoned, or even buzzed, instead of getting shit faced drunk or so high you're helpless, and you have to keep taking it further, and further, go to therapy. Recovery can work, but it starts with you.

If you want to do drugs recreationally, party, have a good time, follow these ten golden rules. They can save you and your life. They can save you heartache and headache. If you want to be a drug dealing kingpin baller who's rolling in the dough and dope, you need to know the way things currently are, especially with this current mantra of violence as an all-in-one problem solver and business solution, everything you earn or procure will be temporary.

If you find yourself in an unfortunate situation where you need medication for long term quality of life, but especially medication that has the potential to be addictive, you need to check yourself and take personal responsibility. If you are a medical provider, don't withhold medication. It is unethical to allow your patients to suffer, especially when you still get paid after you refuse to help with a patient's pain. Instead, learn how to check your patients and teach them to check themselves. If you're a patient, there may, and probably will, come a point that you think you aren't getting the beneficial properties from your medication(s) that you once were. In most cases, (antidepressants and more than a few others aside) what has really happened is your tolerance has reached a point where it knows how to cope with the drugs in your system. What you are actually experiencing is a lack of the high those same medications once so amply provided. You still have the pain killing properties of the drug, or the anxiety relieving properties, or the muscle relaxing abilities, etc. It is simply harder to recognize that because up until now, the high has been the telltale sign that your medication is doing its job, has started working, or has worn off. This is the ideal place where your medical providers want you. So that you have the extra relief you need, but you are still mentally functional. Is it an ideal situation? Absolutely not. For someone who is disabled and in pain on a permanent basis, that high might be the only reason some of us are still alive. "Yeah, I'm miserable, but at least I get these little breaks." It's similar to breaking a pain flare-up pattern by providing temporary relief through trigger point injections. They aren't really going to fix anything except breaking the cycle of pain, which makes it easier and sometimes that is what is needed to even make it possible to get a pain flare-up pattern under control. Same with severe depression. You periodically need a catalyst, like using dynamite to clear a rockslide from a mountain road. And I'm not referring to antidepressants as the dynamite but as the rockslide that blocks your road of life from making further progress.

This is where medication sabbaticals come into play. The status quo for way too long has been that when your medications no longer worked (or seemed like that because the high part is gone), take more, increase dosage, and/or increase strength. I've heard it from almost every single medical provider that I have seen. "When this medication stops working, the only choice is to increase your dosage or switch to taking a stronger medication." This methodology only leads to one place, addiction. Addiction leads to only two places, premature death and/or jail, if you don't catch yourself and possibly need to get sober. However, if you take a sabbatical instead of taking more, you now have an opportunity to gauge how much pain/discomfort you are still in. If you switch to only taking over-the-counter pain medications during this time (if you can), it will give you a window into life without those prescription medications and the amount of relief they really provided compared to over-the-counter pain relievers. During a sabbatical, if you're really honest with yourself (and you need to be), it can help you determine whether or not you can do without it. For some of us, we discover there is no choice. We need the strong subsets of medications and thus the only actual choice is the necessity to learn how to control it. During a sabbatical, you also have the opportunity to listen for cravings. The kind of craving that says "addicted." Take this seriously and honestly. If you crave it, if you want it, if you feel like you can't live without it, let alone turn it down, take note. It will feel like a pull, like an irresistible draw. If you do feel it, stop taking it, get help, and possibly never go back. This will be a much different sensation than the uncomfortable feeling you will have when flushing anything from your system that your body has become accustomed to. For some, a sabbatical can also serve as a learning curve. It can give perspective that this is how much you will hurt or suffer if you abuse your medication and get cut off, blacklisted. A lot of people think that street drugs are an acceptable alternative if they do end up getting out of control and eventually get cut off from a medical provider's help. They are not. But desperate people in desperate situations do desperate things, and I personally cannot blame you.

Again, make no mistake, when taking a medication sabbatical, your body will revolt a little. This is not necessarily an addiction. This is simply your body becoming adjusted to not having what it has become accustomed to. It can happen with anything you take or consume on a regular basis, to varying degrees. Stop drinking your morning coffee, you're going to be a little miserable for a few days. Probably with daily afternoon headaches for a week or so, perhaps some constipation, and let's not forget irritability and feeling a bit more tired than usual. Cutting sugar out of your diet? Get ready for your body to express displeasure. Changing or discontinuing some antidepressants, things will get very uncomfortable. But again, these aren't addictions. An addiction is like I described in the previous paragraphs and chapters. If you wean off and discontinue your opioid painkillers, again your body will revolt a bit but as long as you aren't in a craving situation or longing for the high, you're not experiencing signs of being addicted.

I would also imply that when a patient has a vast array of adverse reactions to varying classifications of medications, such as myself, the typical and newer alternatives to opioid pain management are probably not a good or viable option. Even a minor adverse reaction can be horrible, but a severe adverse reaction is devastating. And going that route is asking for trouble by increasing the chances of varying and unforeseen adverse reactions in more, and more, patients.

You can also take a mini sabbatical to gain perspective by skipping a day here and a day there, while paying attention to your discomfort level. Simply by lessening your dosage for an extended period of time and eventually going back to full daily dosage.

You need and should wean off and discontinue your medications for a short time, and periodically, not only to check yourself, but so you can also see that they are still helping you (or if they are not, take appropriate action), and thus you also lower your tolerance level. Now, when you restart your medications or go back to full dosage, it will work more like it did, and now you don't need stronger, more potentially addictive medication. When you restart your medication, you get that mental break as well. It's okay to laugh because you are high, and it's okay to get high to do that, again within reason. Or you can continue to take it on a regiment and benefit from the extra pain killing properties without the high part. As long as you can keep the perspective that it is still helping you and your pain, as well as other ailments, that would all be so much worse without it. When you discontinue a prescription, if you find out that it wasn't helping you at all or even that it may have been hurting you, take appropriate action by not taking that medication (or medications) anymore. Even if you need to wean off of them to do it.

If you want to start from scratch, or close to it, you can completely clean your system out. Wean off and discontinue your medications, and do a light flushing regiment of hot soaks, preferably with Epsom salts, and drink a lot of water, until your chemical side effects subside, and you are only dealing with your actual medical ailments, after that, you can restart your medications. You can even restart them one at a time, to make sure your medications are, in fact, more beneficial than harmful.

Or you can wait for one of those forced sabbaticals when the doctor's office didn't manage to get your refill in before a long holiday break. Or the pharmacy failed to get your medications reordered. Or your medications were recalled for safety reasons. And if you do partake in recreational substances that are illegal, let's call getting busted a forced sabbatical, take advantage of it.

Aside from a sabbatical for perspective, and improving how well your medications/drugs work, a good way to teach yourself control, or teach your patients control with taking potentially addictive medications is to get a pill box. One that has thirty-days' worth of medication boxes. As soon as you, the patient, gets a prescription/refill you load your pill box (a one or two week pill box will work as well, you will just need to refill it more often. In each of the thirty-day boxes you put in one day's worth of medications. That is how many, for example, painkillers and muscle relaxers you have allotted for that day. Again, just for an easy example, let's say four-10 milligram Vicodin/hydrocodone (an opioid painkiller) and four-10 milligram Soma/carisoprodol (a muscle relaxer) to get you through each twenty-four-hour period.

Each one of those boxes contains enough medication for you to get by in a twenty-four-hour period. That's get by, not be so freaking high you can't even feel that you're lying on the television remote, let alone feel your pain. No, in most reasonable cases, that's enough pain relief that you're no longer in agony but you are still aware of your physical limits, and you're mentally aware of your surroundings, as well as being semi-functional (medical issues excluded). That might mean still tolerating a small amount of pain and discomfort but tolerating exponentially less pain than if you were only taking Tylenol/acetaminophen (an ingredient already present in a lot of narcotic painkillers) and even still, way less pain than if you were taking nothing at all. That way you can remain at least a little aware of your existing pain, so you don't make anything you already deal with worse.

Now for only a moment, let's imagine that you took all eight of those pills first thing in the morning. The four painkillers and the four muscle relaxers. You figured, "I'm going to get total relief for just a little while." About five to six hours later, those medications that you took improperly begin to wear off. Now you have about eighteen hours of elevated, and even extreme, agony to contend with, or you can take just one or two out of another day. But if you do that, then you have a day or two in the future where you have less, and less medication, and most likely, eventually none at all. Because you misused your medication, as you mistakenly thought complete pain relief now was better than eighty or ninety percent of partial ailment relief all the time. The more you take medications ahead of when you were supposed to, the more severe and longer that your suffering will eventually be.

Whereas, if you treat each box that has a day's worth of medication as prescribed, you can make it through the day (and the month) with minimal difficulties and with as much control over your symptoms as possible. The more you practice this, the sooner you will come to realize that maybe you could wait an hour or two to take that next dose. Eventually, that leads to skipping a whole dose all together, but only occasionally. Which should be the goal. Being adequately medicated means it is available when you need it, with the absence of abuse, so that occasionally you won't need to take full dosage throughout the day, allowing you to come up with an extra "pill" every now and again. At this point, when you do have that day of extra pain, for whatever reason, or you need to break that pain flare-up cycle that your normal regiment can't get a hold of, you now have that extra "pill" to help you accomplish exactly that, and without causing a problem. And you can now also do so, as you have successfully learned, and demonstrated that you can take the medication that you need with responsibility.

The idea of staying ahead of chronic pain is only correct when you learn what it takes to control your pain. Not taking pain medications, or let's say anxiety pills, or even muscle relaxers on a set concrete regiment, no matter what, indiscriminately. You need to learn how to stay ahead of your pain, yes, but you also need to learn how to take advantage of those situations where you are able to skip a dose. I would argue that taking pain medications every day, no matter what, on a regiment, like a robot, will lead to an addiction quicker, rather than skipping the occasional dose for the simple fact that you listened to your body and realized that you didn't need another dose right then, hence you didn't take a pill simply because it was time. Even if you had a day when you were able to take your medications every eight hours instead of every six, right there, you came up with an emergency dose for one of those bad days in the future, when the limits of a regiment of maintenance doesn't cut it, or allow for that much need, occasional extra dosage.

I'd also love to tell you that all I need to do to manage my ailments is take pills. This is also a great misconception. There is no such thing as a miracle medication or drug, marijuana included. Learning how to manage your medication is, in fact, only step one in successfully managing any ailment. This is also another way that I have managed to keep my dosage low. As I mentioned, a painkiller should mitigate a good portion of your pain, but not all of it. You need to utilize other pain management tools as well. For example, I use physical therapy, stretches, self-adjustments, heat pads, ice packs, and various muscle creams. Hot tubs and/or Epsom salt soaks have been paramount for my ailments to be under control. Along with various other pain control techniques, like the mitigation of pain by treating trigger points with pressure, also known as acupressure. Different distractions can also be useful. I've always believed that everyone should have a hobby. Like a legit hobby, not exterminating walking digital mushrooms and disgruntled tech turtles as a colorful plumber in a video game.

Unfortunately, there will always be those who do have an inclination for drug abuse that are both medical patients and not medical patients at all. I have two bits of advice for patients dealing with people like this. People referred to as drug seekers. Don't tell anyone what medications you take, and if anyone knows, ask them to keep it to themselves. And keep your medications (even your recreational dope) locked up. Keep in mind that a locked door, drawer, or even a padlock doesn't keep anyone from stealing from you. A lock does however have the potential to keep honest people honest. As well as having the potential as another check for yourself to keep from taking an extra pill. The act of having to get your keys and unlock the drawer they are in, gives you that extra time to consider, "Do I need an extra pill, or am I just seeking an extra thrill?"

Prescribing newer pain alternatives, like Wellbutrin or Suboxone, as opposed to the more traditional pain medications, like a traditional opioid based painkiller, for example hydrocodone or oxycodone, is proving to be a worse outcome. The side effects, especially long-term, are worse in most of these cases. Medications that prescribers have deemed safe, patients are getting high on them, in a worse way than the drugs they are supposed to replace, as a result, people are now starting to drug seek them as well. The narrative needs to change. When you have a need for a painkiller on a temporary basis to help you get through some initial acute pain, the narrative needs to be more than, "you need to watch yourself, this medication can be highly addictive." You need to tell your patient what the draw of an addiction feels like. You need to tell the patient, and the patient needs to understand, that it doesn't matter how much you like or enjoy the feeling of this painkiller (or any other medication that can be addictive), it is a temporary situation, and as such, once the acute part of their pain is over, so is the use of painkillers. They need to know and accept that. When someone leaves a hospital and decides they liked the high of morphine or fentanyl so much they want it again and they go find and do it, that's when people really get into the downward spiral of addiction. When they do indeed keep taking more to keep getting high and eventually just to feel better, not good, just better. Any substance that has a near unbreakable and irresistible pull like that should never be indulged in the first place. But not all drugs are like that, despite the stigma. Oh, and the argument that opioid painkillers are not intended for long term use as they were never tested for long term, is one-hundred percent bullshit. And that goes double anytime a medical professional makes this argument with any medication. As in, no medication is tested for long term use until after it is released to the public for approved use. From that point on, is where long term testing begins and continues. It is far from a scientific approach and is solely based on observation.

If you're in the unfortunate situation of needing prescription painkillers, or any variety of other medications that come with an intoxication side effect warning, and there are so many medications that do, again you need to understand that side effect of intoxication should not be used as a gauge of whether or not your medication is still working. Whether or not the last dosage you took has kicked in or is currently wearing off. You need to pay attention to your pain, ailments, and discomfort level instead. Especially if you're taking medication that is newer on the market. At that point, and in that instance, you are one of the first long-term, drug testing guinea pigs for that new drug/medication.

If you're in chronic, constant pain, and you are new or newish at taking medications, you have surely noticed that you're still aware of at least a portion of your pain, but you convince yourself that it's not so bad because of the "high." Convincing yourself that the "high" is a nice distraction from the pain, is only that, a distraction and you need to realize that the intoxication part is not really killing or alleviating any actual pain. If you were to forgo your medication, maybe skip a single dose, or even take a short sabbatical, or even end up taking your next dosage late due to unforeseen circumstances, or take a half or even a quarter of your regular dosage for the next two to three days. For the sole purpose of gauging how much pain you are still in, and how much your painkiller, or anxiety medication, or whatever medication is actually still helping you, even without the intoxication part. And if you find out that it's not helping, well, there's no sense in taking medication that you don't need.

When medical providers tell patients that once your tolerance reaches a certain point the only option is to increase your dosage. Which eventually leads to guaranteed addiction on a long enough timeline. Then your patients do develop an addiction, that status quo is to cut them off from quality-of-life medications with the rationalization that, "pain won't kill you." No, it won't, but suffer badly enough, on a long enough timeline, and most people will handle it themselves. As I mentioned, and as we have all seen, even with good decent intelligent people who are also getting hopelessly addicted to street drugs, or alcohol, because they don't want to hurt or suffer anymore, or even worse, commit suicide because they can't take it anymore and from there, from that perspective, it is easy to feel like nobody cares about their pain and suffering. I promise, after someone becomes disabled, they question their value and worth in more ways than you could possibly imagine. Achieving quality of life makes hard medical times bearable. Addiction shouldn't even be a secondary concern in instances like that, but rather fifth, or maybe even tenth on the concern list, if considered at all, especially for the more extreme cases of suffering.

I believe that less is more, and medications, addictive medications, but especially opioid painkillers, go a lot further than most realize. I was once told that the reason the medical field likes fentanyl so much is it is both a painkiller and a sedative. Sometimes patients on strong IV painkillers, like morphine, will become violent or even uncontrollable. On fentanyl, no one is belligerent and out of control. Simply because the high is so intense you can't do anything, let alone voice your opinion. Forget fighting back. It makes you have a feeling that is similar to your body and mind floating in water. That combination of painkillers and sedatives is also why it is so addictive. For years now, we have known and warned against combining medications like that and given the outcome for people who get in trouble with fentanyl, it doesn't seem like it is a better option, even if it comes from a prescription pad, hospital, or pharmacy. And if we're being honest, the medical community prefers to start on that level, out of an abundance of convenience. Convenience for them. It is not convenient for the medical patient that leaves the hospital with a nearly hopeless addiction. Maybe only consider using drugs like fentanyl in extreme last case scenario situations? But please keep in mind this suggestion is coming from a patient who has been inconvenienced. Not a medical provider seeking convenience in their practice.

Once again, for chronic pain patients like me who unfortunately need medications that have the potential for addiction, as there is no better option for our situation, I would not only suggest but strongly recommend periodic sabbaticals. For three reasons, you can check yourself for signs of addiction, you can appropriately gauge your level of pain, unencumbered by medications, and you can reset your tolerance. This will tell you if you still need your medications, how well they were, and are still working for you, even if you didn't realize it at the time. As well as let you know if you are becoming reliant on them, in more than a medical necessity kind of way. And if you discover that you still need them and you aren't becoming addicted, now your tolerance has been reset. Now you don't need an increase in medications, dosage strength, nor frequency. When I first started to take sabbaticals, I really thought I was doing better than I was. What was actually happening, I had become complacent on my medications, not realizing my pain was still really high, until I didn't have the pain blocking properties of said medications. That was a wake-up call for me that a lot of patients need.

Fortunately, and unfortunately, the best diagnostic tool for a medical provider is the patient's personal experience. Fortunately, because that's the person you're trying to help. It's the equivalent of a car being able to talk to an automobile mechanic, or a dog having a verbal conversation with their veterinarian. Unfortunately, a medical provider cannot feel what you feel, patients can sometimes have ulterior motives, and sometimes medical providers aren't trusting enough. I get it, people can lie, and people can tell the truth, so how do you tell them apart? A question that I cannot answer. And a problem that needs a fool proof solution, and it would solve a lot of problems in the medical world, and hence society as well. For me, I never would have walked into a doctor's office if I didn't need the help that only they can provide, of which, most of the time, I have not received anything past the bare minimum. Better than nothing, right? It is, until you consider how unethical it can be for anyone to be paid for a job that you can't even do, but one that you also can't identify. And I get that too; there's a reason it's called "practicing medicine." But if we're being honest, that has become another go-to answer for medical providers. Instead of what it really is, an excuse, a rationalization, a justification. That needs to stop, and some semblance of an actual work ethic needs to be established in the medical field. Again, work all the hours that you want, if you can't finish the job, you still lack a work ethic.

And a note on over medicating and writing off-label medications. At a certain point, this too needs to stop. Doctors can start throwing chemical drugs at a patient's ailments, to see what sticks, and when this happens it is guess work. It is the equivalent of throwing darts at a dart board, in a darkened bar, after spinning around until you're dizzy, while also being blindfolded. You're probably not even going to hit the same wall the dart board is on.

I have a hypothesis for the medical community. If a patient can handle taking prescription opioid painkillers until they are put on an antidepressant, did the patient really have a problem with the opioids, or did the anti-depressants cause the problem by modifying the patient's brain chemistry in unexpected ways? And if that patient later manages to get off their antidepressants, and is once again, able to demonstrate that they can and are able to handle the rigors of taking something with the potential for addiction, which medication was the real problem? My hypothesis is, if a patient is cut-off from their painkillers while at the same time taking brain altering antidepressants, and they didn't have any of those "addict" problems before taking antidepressants, and other patients who only take painkillers, have no issue whatsoever, or even less issues, which is the real problem?

The Real Monsters in the Medicine Cabinet

Marijuana is one of the most useful, least harmful, wonderfully versatile all natural medications, as long as it is used responsibly and within reason. Like anything and everything, moderation is paramount. Alcohol is also okay with extreme moderation. Nicotine in any form, not okay. If you are in the unfortunate situation of needing medication for quality of life, less is more. Always remember to listen to your body, and if your medical provider isn't listening to you, get ready to stand up for yourself or prepare to get fucked. Or get a new medical provider that does listen. The job of a medical provider is to listen, evaluate, diagnose, and then present and explain all of the options available to you, the patient. You, the patient, will then decide on the best course of action for you. Anything outside of those parameters and the medical provider, is being unethical, and all about business, and not actually practicing medicine, but rather participating in profiteering.

When the accumulation of an unreasonable number of injuries and accidents finally caught up with me at the age of twenty-six, they also led me right to the middle of being way over-medicated. With thirteen different medications running amuck in my system, I was way too high. Even the people around me noticed. One day my mother, of all people, came to me and said, "I would rather you smoke a little pot than take extra pills." It didn't take long to think about what she said. She had a profound point. It was, in fact, one of those slaps in the face epiphanies that I should've already had. So, I took her advice as much as I could. But because it was still illegal, my marijuana use was limited to piece meal situations, and dependent on whether my friends had any as well as how generous and compassionate they were feeling. Which meant I was still largely reliant on pharmaceuticals for quality of life. In 2010, when medical marijuana became legal in Colorado, it opened a whole world of better possibilities. For myself and everyone else, as well. Now marijuana is in such a readily available supply that it can be taken like medication, on a regiment. I went from feeling like a pharmacy junkie, a pseudo smack addict, to regaining my mental faculties after eventually replacing more than a few prescriptions. Had I not had that opportunity, the plethora of medications I was on, would have killed me. No ifs, ands, or buts about it.

As I previously mentioned, drug use is no fairy tale, and it would be unbalanced, unwise, and unfair of me to fail to mention the casualties of drug use that I have seen. That has been a part of, and affected, my life and the people I know, and care for.

Let's start with my last girlfriend, Cindy. In high school Cindy was one of the most beautiful and popular girls. She was also an exceptional vocalist. As such, she would often be asked to sing our national anthem at many local events. She eventually developed pancreatitis and was also diagnosed with chronic pain along with a few other things. She struggled with her vast array of symptoms for a very long time, never really finding the relief she so desperately needed. One day her doctor prescribed her two different medications that should never be taken in tandem, let alone prescribed together. The pharmacist also failed to catch it. Trusting in her medical providers, she took them both as instructed, went to bed, and never woke up. She left behind two children, a little boy at the age of seven, and a little girl at the age of four.

Two years before that, I lost my friend Matty. Matty and I had been good friends since kindergarten. He was one of the first people I reconnected with when I first came back to my small hometown. He conned me out of some pills to get high, under the guise that his back hurt and he couldn't get the help he needed. I quickly caught on and told him I wouldn't give him anymore, thinking that would be the end of it. Instead, he went bar surfing until he came across a gal by the name of Jessica. Jessica was one of many patients of Dr. Duplicitous, our local pill mill doctor who eventually got busted along with his partner. Rumor was that if all you wanted were pills, go see Dr. Duplicitous and simply tell him what you want. Jessica didn't like the way medications made her feel, so she used the prescriptions he wrote for her, as a source of extra income. She sold Matty methadone, percocet, vicodin, xanax, ativan, and a few others. A while before this, Matty said to me one day, "The way my mind works, if one pill feels good, then ten should feel great!"

I looked him right in the eyes and said, "Matty, that's overdose level." He scoffed and refused to even consider my advice. After his sister found his cold body lying lifeless on his couch, autopsy revealed so many ill-gotten medications in his system that his family had to convince the coroner that he wasn't suicidal at all, and it was, in fact, unintentional. Anyone who knew him could tell you he was an incredibly jovial individual and had no reason or desire to commit suicide. Now, I blame Matty for taking those pills and ignoring my advice, but I also blame that doctor for putting profits above patients. Matty wasn't the only person he killed. I also blame Jessica for deciding to put profits over another human being's life. She and her pill mill provider are murderers, convicted or not.

During high school I had two good friends, we hung out most of the time. So close, and such good friends, I often considered us three amigos or even three musketeers. They both tried meth for the first time, at the same time I did. And they have both struggled with severe addictions and all the horrors that come with it, for the last twenty-five years, give or take. Once again, I will mention that I was an anomaly, a chance happening, that I got lucky through a fluke happening, where they did not.

While in the process of writing this book, I ran into another very old, very good friend that I have had the pleasure of knowing since the first grade. Jack had recently lost his wife and unborn child. She had experienced a severe adverse reaction to the antidepressant she was on during her pregnancy. It caused her to take her own life along with the life of her unborn son. Jack said that he went to her last mental health appointment with her, to be supportive, and see if they could get her depression straightened out, as the antidepressant she was on was making things worse. He told me how they both expected her psychiatrist to take her off that medication due to the horrible time she was having with it. He looked me right in the eyes and said, "I was holding her hand as her doctor said he was going to increase her dosage, instead of taking her off it. Grant, I literally felt her give up. It was like I could feel her give up, like all hope instantly drained from her body, when he said that." A knot began to develop in my chest out of grief for what my friend and his wife experienced. That horrible knot quickly grew and morphed into an even larger feeling of despair. I could've sworn it felt like a simple square knot but became more akin to a Gordon's Knot the moment he filled in the rest of the blanks. The exact same medical provider that hurt me with antidepressants, in the exact same clinic, with the exact same drug.

I would love to tell you that if any drug has medicinal value, it can only help. Just like any drug that is illegal doesn't have any medicinal value. It is simply not the case. My friends and I noticed something while we were growing up and being wild teenagers. Anytime we would trip hallucinogens, especially acid (L.S.D.), or mushrooms (psilocybin), our moods and mental state would be elevated for months at a time. Now, that trick is being studied with mushrooms, ketamine, and L.S.D. along with a few others, but those are the main three. My personal experience tells me that mushrooms are probably the safest route, with benefits that will last longer than ketamine, with less side effects. L.S.D. will give the longest lasting mental benefits, as long as you don't flip out and lose it, which is an actual possibility. If someone can figure out why some people are never the same after tripping acid once, and why some people can trip on and off for their whole lives and never have a problem, then and only then will L.S.D. be a more viable and safer medication.

I don't know about you, but if I had to choose between taking an antidepressant or two everyday along with a medication or two to negate the side effects of my antidepressants, only to have to find a new antidepressant or increase dosage every few years, versus tripping acid once or twice a year, with zero lasting negative side effects, I already know which one I would choose. As far as the ketamine option goes, I have a strong inclination that this one might cause more problems than it helps, down the road. I personally lost two friends that wanted to try tripping acid and never came all the way back after they did. And no, they didn't spend the rest of their lives believing they were an airplane or thinking they were a glass of orange juice. Instead, it triggered bipolar disorder in one of them and schizophrenia in the other. If you're going to try those routes, proceed with caution and godspeed.

If I had to tell you which drugs are okay, and which ones aren't, this is what you should pay attention to. As long as moderation can be practiced, it is more than likely okay to indulge in. That means drugs such as methamphetamines, heroin, PCP, fentanyl, etc. should never be taken. That also includes the new "gas station heroin" known as tianeptine, as well as kratom, and bath salts. If a drug, or herb, is chemically altered for more potency/concentration, it is probably more harmful than you realize. Above all else, listen to your body and mind to make sure whatever you take, medical or recreational, is more helpful than harmful.

If you're a doctor and patients are seeking medication from you that isn't technically intoxicating, they may be getting high on it in unexpected ways. Some antidepressants are sought after for nefarious reasons and enbibed by illicit means. A similar thing is happening with a certain drug that is designed for coming off addictive substances, specifically breaking addictions to opioids, and at the same time it also keeps other opioids from working by blocking their effects on opioid receptors. People are crushing and then snorting the pill or dissolving the gel patches into a solution like a saline solution, then shooting it up. If someone takes a drug, like that, to get high, and it also prevents opioids from working, the only way for an addict to keep getting high is to continue to take that specific drug in unconventional ways, or they can take something that is much, much, stronger. Which we now know is another problem, that leads to another problem, and another. Nothing was solved there and there is a plethora of prescriptions that can be abused like this, not just these few examples. I do apologize for being vague. In my experience it is better not to tell someone how to open Pandora's Box.

I could keep giving examples, but along with my personal and horrific experiences with certain medications that I have already shared, I believe I have made my point. That no drug is safe and it is high time to acknowledge the limitations of mankind's ability to manufacture chemical compounds that make up modern day pharmaceuticals, and the sometimes severe and debilitating drawbacks of many pharmaceuticals' side effects that often multiply and compound with each other.

It is also time that we expand our horizons and gaze beyond the constraints of modern medicine. I'm not saying scrap medications and western medicine all together, I'm saying we need to cure, not treat. If medical drugs can't do that, maybe a little help from mother nature is what the doctor ordered. And if our bodies naturally have cannabinoid receptors and opioid receptors, it is logical that, when these medications are consumed, manufactured, and/or grown correctly, that they might actually be far more beneficial, and way less harmful, instead of something else that also gets us high, or alters brain chemistry in unexpected ways because it doesn't belong in our bodies?

At a certain point a medical patient's best option becomes mitigation of ailments rather than curing the cause. I believe this has become common practice and a go-to, that like antidepressants, should be the very last course of action. I'm not saying this isn't necessary for some. I'm saying when the success rate of the medical field is helping less people than the failures and shortcomings of modern medicine are hurting, it's time for an occupational enema.

If you are seemingly hopelessly addicted, you have three basic options. Get sober and never touch any intoxicating substance again. This may be your only option. Especially if any time you become intoxicated, buzzed, or stoned, it triggers you to want a bigger, better, or even a badder high. Or, if you can wrap your mind around only using marijuana and come to terms with that type and level of high is as good as it gets. At that point you can not only get stoned, but you can also utilize marijuana to help you break the hold of a highly addictive substance. I've seen three different people use marijuana to aid them in the cessation of their specific addictions. That's two alcoholics, and one meth addict, that are no longer addicts, and function as productive members of society, while currently using and enjoying marijuana with moderation. Or option number three, do nothing, remain on the same hopeless, dead-end track, and end up incarcerated, prematurely embalmed, or worse.

I truly hope that anyone who reads my book finds the help or solace they need. If you found my book and ideas offensive, I would ask, did you read it with an open mind? Or were you simply looking for a fight? As no offense was intended. This is the solution no one has come up with yet. As well as the constructive criticism, the medical field needs to go beyond the current limitation of the industry. From one person, out of many, that was never asked how to fix it but should have been the first group of people to be consulted. The only ones who matter, the ones who have taken medications, the patients. The ones who have the firsthand perspective. The ones who have done the drugs, taken the medications, and not ruined their life. And now you should not only know that it is possible, but necessary.

My Own Rule Enumeration (or M.O.R.E.)

A few lines for M.O.R.E. things you may learn along the way

My Own Rule Enumeration (or M.O.R.E.)

A few lines for M.O.R.E. things you may learn along the way

My Own Rule Enumeration (or M.O.R.E.)

A few lines for M.O.R.E. things you may learn along the way

Bibliography

More by the author...

We shall see...

About the Author

Even though there is more to know about me, what more can I say about myself that my book hasn't? Too much more might be predominantly preposterous, pruning the purpose of this parchment. So, I will leave you with this perfunctory prologue…

Born and raised in Colorado, I had always thought and hoped for a life of creativity, which I enjoy so much, but from a very young age there was always work to be done. Even though it seemed at times inconvenient, it taught me many valuable life lessons. Through a series of many unfortunate events and a few merciful miracles, I gained perspective through my suffering, as well as from what I was spared. One day it was made clear to me that I needed to share what I have learned with the rest of the world. After some encouraging words from a close friend, I began to write my first book, this book. Transforming the harsh lessons and copious sufferings of my life into productive literary creativity, that can hopefully help others. Besides, even if it ends up only telling a good story, even stories have value.

www.ingramcontent.com/pod-product-compliance
Lightning Source LLC
LaVergne TN
LVHW090515110826
845146LV00003B/869

* 9 7 9 8 9 9 3 6 7 1 3 1 4 *